The Therapeutic Power of Herbal Gardening

DISCOVER HIGHLY-EFFECTIVE MEDITATIVE PATHS TO OPTIMAL HOLISTIC HEALTH

LES PIERRE

Contents

Introduction: The Healing Haven of Herbal Gardening

Seeking a healthy habit that fits your busy schedule while providing many benefits? Thinking of infusing your living space with a sense of calm and peacefulness or a touch of nature? What if I told you that the simple, science-backed practice of herbal gardening could provide you with all these advantages and so much more? Imagine building your herbal garden, a personal healing haven designed to fit your individual needs, giving you all the inherent tranquility that comes with gardening and, with the guidance of this book, the ability to craft your natural healing remedies or brew your rejuvenating herbal teas. With the power of fresh herbs readily available in the comfort of your home, there's no end to the holistic possibilities.

Herbs, with their vibrant colors and enticing aromas, serve purposes far beyond their aesthetic or culinary appeal. With a bit of careful, heartfelt nurturing and a touch of understanding, an herb can offer powerful medicinal and therapeutic relief from the burdens of daily life. And with a garden full of these handy plants, you'll have all you need to create powerful remedies for your daily ailments. Imagine a collection of tinctures, oils, ointments, and teas refined from plants you've grown to fight the problems you face. Digestion troubles? Steep some fresh peppermint leaves in hot water for a cup of tea to ease discomfort and soothe stomach aches. Anxiety over a big project at work? Infuse a bit of lemon balm to uplift your mood. Give the health of your hair and scalp a boost with a rosemary rinse, known for its strengthening properties. For soothing benefits on the skin, try using marigold in a carrier oil or adding the petals to a hot bath. The world of herbs is replete with natural pathways to enhance your well-being. And with some knowledge of herbal infusions, the limit is only your imagination.

As we embark on this path of herbal gardening, it is vital to remember that we are not merely cultivating a patch of earth. This journey is about nurturing a space where your garden grows in tandem with your spirit and well-being. This is your sanctuary, a personal retreat where each plant holds the potential for healing your body and mind. It's an oasis where gardening transcends being a simple act of planting, pruning, and harvesting and becomes a holistic practice that boosts your health and tranquility.

Whether you've been gardening for years or decided to try it upon picking up this book, there's always something new and enlightening to discover on your journey to herbal gardening. That's right, no experience is necessary. This path is about cultivating an alternative lifestyle that embraces the healing touch of nature and brings balance and wellness to your life, regardless of your age, career, status, or position in life. If you seek to enhance your life, this path is for you, and we are here to help.

In weaving personal anecdotes throughout, such as the invaluable lessons on herbal gardening bestowed upon me by my late grandmother in my youth, we highlight the deep, meditative connection between our minds and the natural world. My grandmother, with her wisdom and gentle guidance among the fragrant herbs of our backyard garden, instilled in me a profound appreciation for the earth's nurturance. Her teachings imparted knowledge on cultivating and harvesting herbs and how these practices could ground and center us, offering peace amidst life's chaos.

In this guide, we'll examine herbal remedies from a historical perspective and review some of their validated scientific studies, laying a solid foundation for our journey. We'll then guide you through building your herbal arsenal, a collection of plants that are pleasing to the eye and powerful in their healing capabilities. We'll also share practical tips for cultivating a diverse herbal garden, nurturing your soil and soul, and harvesting the energy of seasonal herbs.

You'll also learn to create sacred spaces and integrate herbs into meditation practices. We'll advise you on how to craft herbal elixirs for emotional resilience and transform living spaces into green havens utilizing herbs' wellness and tranquil properties. We'll give you a few tips for sustainable practices and help you understand the crucial role of herb advocacy in the broader community.

Each herb in your garden tells its unique story, a narrative of healing and rejuvenation. We'll explore how tending to these plants becomes meditative, fostering a profound and nurturing connection between your mind and the natural world. We weave personal narratives and case studies throughout the story, illustrating the transformative impact of a mindful herbal garden. These stories showcase how individuals have achieved mental clarity, stress relief, and a more profound sense of peace through their gardening endeavors.

To enhance your journey, we've included a handy Note Pad section for jotting down your homemade recipes and personal garden insights, making your experience with this book genuinely personal. This guide aims to inform and inspire. We'll point you in the right direction to not only teach you but to help you grow as well. We believe that even if you read casually, there's always something new and enlightening to discover on your journey through herbal gardening.

So, let us uncover the secrets of holistic healing through the magic of an herbal garden and begin or continue transforming our living spaces into vibrant sanctuaries of health and serenity.

CHAPTER 1
The Roots of Healing

Let us begin our journey with a story on the transformative power of herbal living. Lily Hamilton spoke with us about her first apartment and the overwhelming emotions she experienced when she first saw it as a college student in a new town. The moment she walked in, the room's faded, peeling wallpaper, lonely, dust-covered floors, and plain counters brought her to tears. The space made her anxious that she could never make it feel like home, and she feared she would be miserable. However, Lily found solace in a classmate named Lashawn, who, soon after their meeting, became one of her closest friends. Lashawn invited Lily to her small apartment for a party, and Lily was amazed by what she saw. Despite its smaller size, Lashawn's apartment was a joy. It was filled with unique aromas and beautiful flourishing plants in wall planters and pots by the window. Impressed by Lashawn's green oasis, Lily asked her for advice on achieving a similar atmosphere in her place. Lashawn happily visited Lily's house, and within a few weeks, Lily's apartment transformed into a vibrant sanctuary with herbs growing in the garden, home, and even on the walls. The ease and fun of herbal gardening thrilled Lily so much she started making her own shampoo and essence oils. The invigorating feeling of gardening can and does spark joy and happiness. No matter the space, a bit of green can work wonders in your home and your heart.

ANCIENT WISDOM MEETS MODERN SCIENCE

We'll start with a brief look back for some historical reference. If something is worth our time, we should know its history. This is especially important should we desire to grow herbs and craft them into remedies. A medicinal herb is only as good as its source and the science to back it. We'll vet the scientific aspects of this growing and harvesting herbs for medicinal purposes, ensuring that these remedies have been tested and are safe for use. But more importantly, we will give you the guidance you'll need to make these assurances as your curiosity and garden grow and thrive. We'll go over a few common remedies you can grow at home, tell you a bit about their history, and provide some insights on them from herbalists all over the globe, both present and past. We need only look to history to learn about the plants we harvest, the properties they contain, and what ailments they can aid.

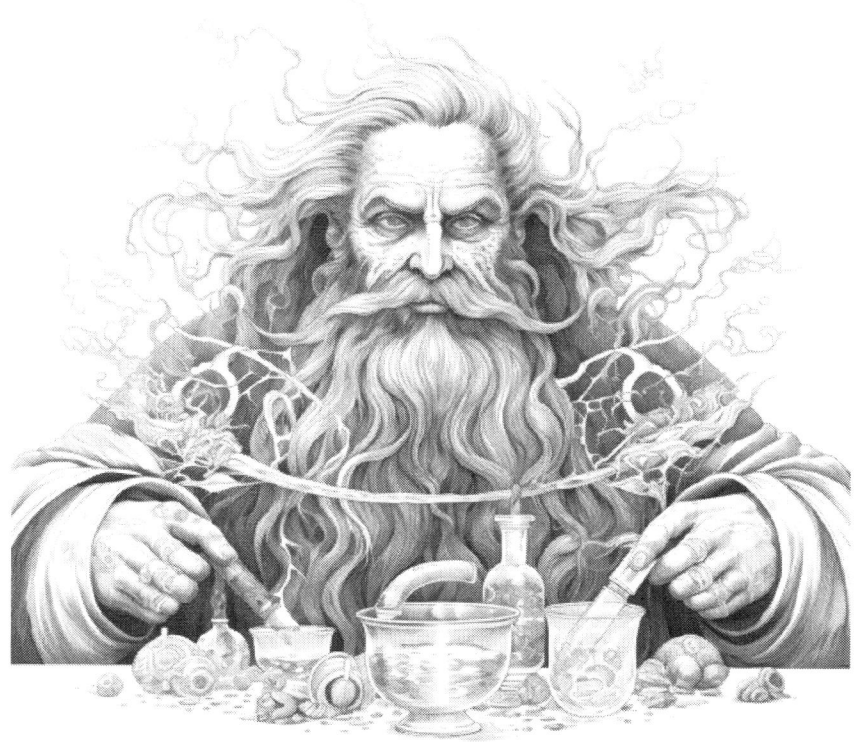

For centuries, herbalists, scientists, and researchers have studied, recorded, and written about herbal medicines. Scholars date the earliest practices of using plants medicinally back thousands of years: "The oldest written evidence of medicinal plants' usage for preparation of drugs has been found on a Sumerian clay slab from Nagpur, approximately 5000 years old. It comprised 12 recipes for drug preparation referring to over 250 various plants" (Petrovska, B. B., 2012).

Taoist philosophy encourages individuals to live in sync with the natural world, fostering a sense of balance and equilibrium. In ancient China, herbal medicine was an art form that aligned with these principles. Practitioners believed that the body was a microcosm of the universe and that herbs could restore balance and promote health. Herbal medicine was about treating physical symptoms and addressing the underlying energetic imbalances in the body. They categorized herbs based on their nature and taste and applied them to restore balance in the body. Ginseng, known as *Ren Shen* in Chinese, was highly valued for its rejuvenating and vitality-boosting properties.

Today, ginseng is a widely recognized supplement, whether found in bottled supplements at a drugstore or infused into popular products like energy drinks. The roots of the ginseng plant are the source of this herbal supplement. Ginseng's journey from the mountainous terrains of China to global popularity is based on its science and history. It has been accepted as a staple of life in our modern society, one we sell in our grocery stores and promote publicly as a known booster of our well-being. So, let's learn a little more about ginseng.

In the comprehensive review titled *Herbal Medicine: Biomolecular and Clinical Aspects*, Wee, Park, and Chung explain that ginseng has a long history of being employed as a folk medicine in East Asian countries. People historically celebrated ginseng as a general tonic and adaptogen, revering it for its ability to maintain the body's resistance to adverse factors and ensure homeostasis. Its applications ranged from improving physical and sexual functions to general vitality and anti-aging.

Modern scientific research has peeled back the layers of this ancient wisdom, revealing the biological activities of ginseng. These studies have shown that ginseng could benefit immunity, cancer, diabetes, CNS functions, and other conditions. The adaptogen properties of ginseng, long observed in traditional practices, are now being validated through scientific inquiry, showcasing its ability to aid the body in maintaining balance and resisting stress.

Building on the legacy of ginseng, let's explore a few more herbal remedies that have withstand the test of time and scientific scrutiny.

Historically, turmeric has been a cornerstone in Ayurvedic medicine for its anti-inflammatory and healing properties. Turmeric, or *Curcuma longa*, has been a staple in Indian cuisine and traditional medicine for centuries. Ancient texts and practices have touted turmeric for its ability to improve digestion, combat infection, and even enhance skin health. In recent years, scientific studies have supported these claims, particularly highlighting curcumin, the active ingredient in turmeric, for its anti-inflammatory effects and potential to treat conditions like arthritis and metabolic syndrome (Prasad S. et al., 2014).

Lavender has been treasured in the Mediterranean for its soothing properties and delightful fragrance. Traditionally, it was used to ease anxiety, insomnia, and depression. Modern research has validated these uses, with studies showing lavender's efficacy in reducing anxiety levels and improving sleep quality, primarily due to its essential oils and active compounds (Koulivand, P. H., et al., 2013).

Echinacea, a native North American plant, is an excellent case study for comparing traditional remedies and scientific findings. Traditionally used by Native American tribes for its immune-boosting and anti-infection properties, echinacea has been the subject of extensive research in the modern era. Numerous studies have indicated that echinacea extracts can enhance immune function, potentially reducing the severity and duration of cold symptoms (Shah, S. A., et al., 2007).

The combination of historical perspectives and scientific validation creates a compelling story in herbal medicine. These examples, from ginseng to echinacea, illustrate a pattern where ancient wisdom is often ahead of its time, waiting for modern science to catch up and provide the empirical evidence that echoes these age-old beliefs.

Herbal remedies, rooted in tradition and validated by science, offer us a unique lens to view health and well-being. As we continue to explore and embrace these natural gifts, we honor the past and contribute to a healthier, more balanced future.

BUILDING YOUR HERBAL ARSENAL

Our research has unearthed the rich histories behind these herbs and the scientific studies that confirm their efficacy. It's clear now that each one brings its distinct advantages. Perhaps you've even learned a few you'd like to equip for your herbal arsenal. If not, don't worry; in this next section, we'll discuss a few of the must-haves we'd suggest for starting your herbal garden and the various ailments they can relieve.

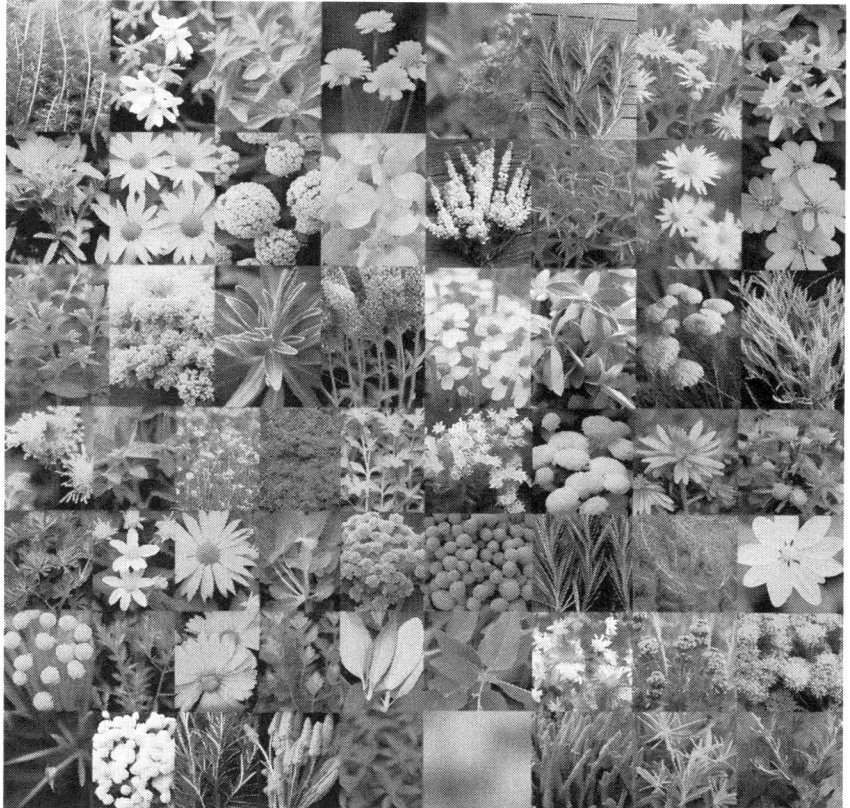

Essential Tools and Herbs for Therapeutic Gardening

In the verdant landscape of herbal gardening, the tools of the trade listed below serve as extensions of the gardener's hands, empowering us to sculpt the fertile canvas of nature's embrace. This section explores the essential tools and techniques that form the backbone of successful herbal cultivation.

3 Tine Pitchfork

A 3 Tine Pitchfork is a garden fork
with three long, pointed prongs or
tines. It is designed with a handle
that can be made of various materials such as wood, fiberglass, or
metal, and the tines are usually
made of sturdy metal to withstand
heavy use. This tool is distin-
guished by its relatively small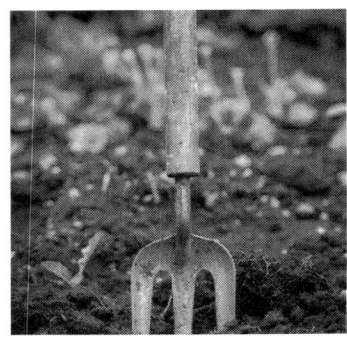
number of tines, often sharp and spaced evenly to optimize its
functionality.

Function

The 3 Tine Pitchfork is versatile and serves multiple purposes in
gardening and agriculture, including:

- **Turning and Aerating Soil**: Its sharp tines are ideal for
  breaking up compacted soil, allowing air and water to
  penetrate more effectively. This improves soil structure
  and promotes healthier root growth.
- **Transplanting**: The pitchfork can lift and move soil
  around young plants or bulbs, making it easier to
  transplant them with minimal damage to the roots.
- **Weeding**: Its pointed tines can get under weeds to lift
  them out of the ground, which is especially useful for
  removing more enormous weeds or those with deep
  roots.
- **Spreading Mulch**: The 3 Tine Pitchfork efficiently
  spreads mulch around plants. Its design allows for easy
  grabbing and scattering of mulch, even in tight spaces.

- **Harvesting Root Vegetables:** This is an effective tool for harvesting root crops like potatoes, carrots, and beets. The tines can loosen the soil around the vegetables, making them easier to pull out without causing damage.
- **Compost Turning:** The pitchfork is also helpful for turning compost piles, helping to aerate the pile and speed up the decomposition process by mixing the materials.

Garden Spade

A spade is a garden tool featuring a long handle and a flat, sharp-edged metal blade. It is designed for digging, cutting through sod and roots, and turning soil.

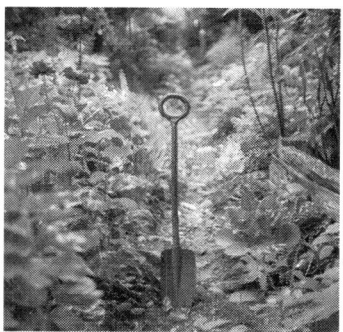

Purpose:

- Digging holes for planting trees, shrubs, and plants.
- Edging beds and borders to create clean lines.
- Turning and aerating soil to prepare garden beds.
- Cutting through tough roots and sod.

Garden Trowel

A trowel is a small hand tool with a pointed, scoop-shaped metal blade and a handle. It is used for digging small holes, transplanting seedlings, and mixing soil or compost.

Purpose:

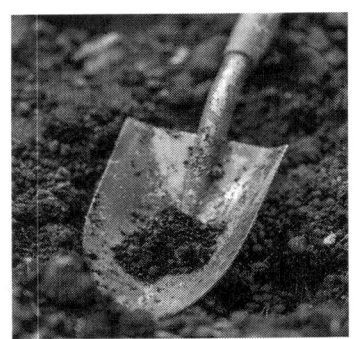

- Planting and transplanting small plants and seedlings.
- Digging small holes for seeds or bulbs.
- Mixing fertilizer or other amendments into the soil.
- Removing weeds around plants.

Pruning Shears

Pruning shears, or hand pruners or secateurs, are scissors for plants designed to cut through branches and stems up to about ¾ inches thick. They typically have sharp blades made of metal and handles that fit comfortably in the hand, often designed to maximize leverage and minimize effort.

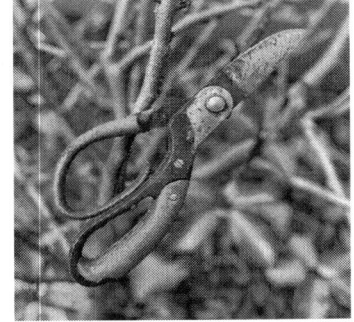

Purpose:

- Pruning dead or overgrown branches and stems to encourage healthy growth and shape plants.
- Deadheading flowers to promote further blooming.
- Cutting back perennials and cleaning up plants during seasonal maintenance.
- Harvesting fruits, vegetables, and cut flowers.

Garden Cart

A garden cart is a wheeled vehicle, often with two or four wheels, designed to transport tools, plants, soil, and other materials across garden terrain.

Purpose:

- Saves time and effort needed to move heavy or bulky items around the garden.
- Increases efficiency in garden tasks by keeping tools and supplies easily accessible.

Gardening Gloves

Gardening gloves are protective coverings designed to fit over the hands. They are made from various materials, such as cotton, leather, rubber, or synthetic blends, and are tailored to offer protection against different gardening hazards.

Purpose:

- Protecting hands from cuts, scrapes, and punctures from thorns, sharp tools, and rough materials.
- Keeping hands clean and dry, preventing soil and sap from staining the skin.
- Providing a better grip on tools, reducing blisters, and improving comfort during extended periods of gardening.
- Protecting hands from harmful chemicals, pests, and irritants in plants and soils.

Moisture Gauge

Definition: A moisture gauge is a tool that measures the amount of water in the soil, helping to prevent over- or under-watering. It typically consists of a probe inserted into the soil to provide a moisture level reading.

Purpose:

- Ensures plants receive the correct amount of water, which is crucial for their health and growth.
- Helps conserve water by indicating when plants need watering, reducing waste.

Soil pH Meter

Definition: A soil pH meter is an instrument used to measure the acidity or alkalinity of the soil. It usually features a probe inserted into the soil, providing a digital or analog reading of the soil's pH level.

Purpose:

- Helps maintain the optimal pH level for plants, ensuring better nutrient uptake and healthier growth.
- Allows for quick adjustments to soil conditions by indicating when to add amendments like lime or sulfur to adjust pH levels.
- I use the Garden Tutor Soil pH Test Strips Kit for my garden. They are usually very accurate and easy to use.
- The kit allows you to place the test strip over the chart for more accurate analysis.

Essential Herbs List

chamomile

- Aids in sleep, anxiety, digestive issues.
- Used in chamomile tea, skin-soothing creams, and calming essential oils.

echinacea

- Aids in immune system boosting, cold and flu prevention.
- Used in immune-boosting teas, tinctures, and throat sprays.

lavender

- Aids in stress relief, insomnia, and skin irritation.
- Used in lavender oil for aromatherapy, relaxing teas, and skincare products.

lemon balm

- Aids in anxiety relief, digestive problems, and insomnia.
- Used in herbal teas, essential oils, and topical ointments for cold sores.

peppermint

- Aids in digestive issues, headaches, and muscle pain.
- Used in peppermint tea, digestive aids, and muscle-soothing balms.

calendula

- Aids in skin conditions, wound healing, and anti-inflammation.
- Used in calendula creams, ointments, and soothing teas.

marshmallow

- Aids in digestive and respiratory issues and skin health.
- Used in herbal teas, cough syrups, and skin care ointments.

thyme (lemon)

- Aids in respiratory infections; antibacterial and antifungal.
- Used in thyme oil, cough remedies, and culinary infusions.

yarrow

- Aids in wound healing, fever reduction, and digestive issues.
- Used in herbal teas, tinctures, and poultices for wounds.

elecampane

- Aids in respiratory conditions like bronchitis and digestive health.
- Used in respiratory tonics, digestive teas, and syrups.

These herbs are readily available in the produce aisle of your local grocery store or within the garden center at your neighborhood hardware store. My grandmother introduced me to cultivating these herbs during my youth, imparting wisdom and techniques I have faithfully adhered to.

Additional Herbs to Consider for Therapeutic Gardening

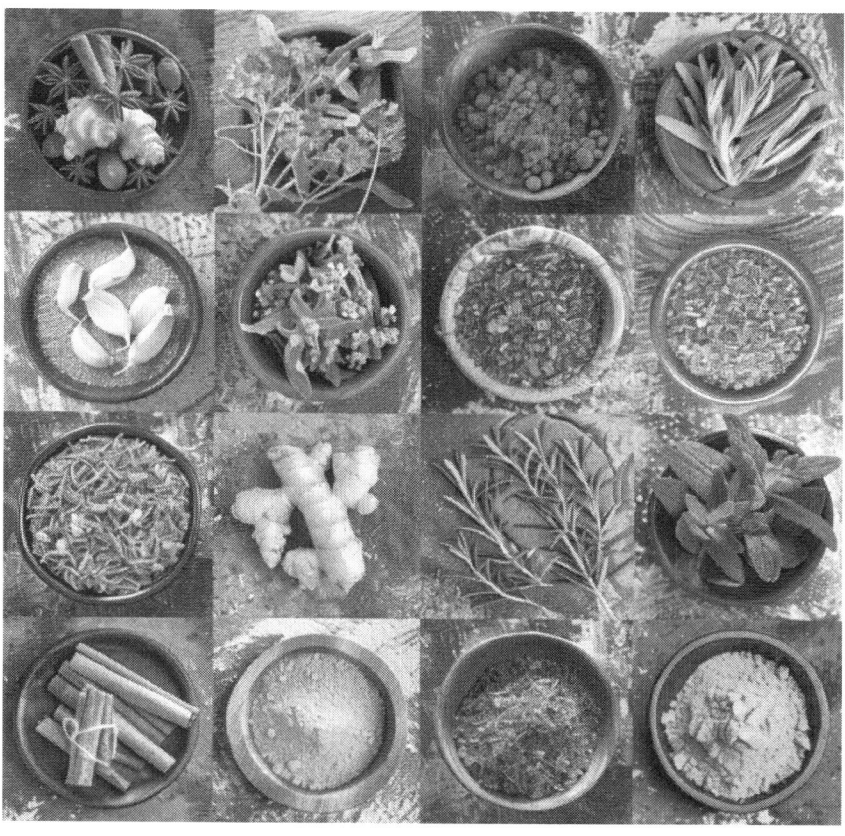

aloe vera

- Soothes skin irritations, aids digestion and supports wound healing.
- The gel extracted from the leaves is applied topically for skin conditions or ingested orally as a juice or supplement.

cayenne

- Supports digestion, improves circulation, and relieves pain.
- Usage: Often used in culinary dishes, as a spice, or capsule form as a supplement.

chickweed

- Soothes skin irritations, supports weight loss, and aids digestion.
- Often consumed as a tea, in salads, or used topically in ointments or poultices.

cinnamon

- It helps regulate blood sugar, reduces inflammation, and fights infections.
- Commonly used in cooking, as a spice, or brewed into teas. Also available in supplement form.

garlic

- Boosts the immune system, lowers blood pressure, and fights infections.
- Usage: Consumed raw, cooked in dishes, or as a supplement in pill form.

ginger

- Eases nausea, aids digestion, and reduces inflammation.
- Often consumed fresh, as a tea, in culinary dishes, or supplement form.

goldenseal

- Fights infections, supports digestive health, and boosts the immune system.
- Often taken in supplement form as capsules or tinctures.

hawthorn

- Supports heart health, regulates blood pressure, and aids digestion.
- Typically consumed as a tea, tincture, or in capsule form.

licorice

- Soothes sore throat, supports adrenal health, and aids digestion.
- Consumed as a tea, in culinary dishes, or taken in supplement form.

mullein

- Supports respiratory health, relieves coughs, and soothes mucous membranes.
- Often brewed into teas, smoked, or used in tincture form.

plantain

- Relieves insect bites, soothes skin irritations, and supports digestive health.
- Leaves can be chewed or made into a poultice for topical application or brewed into teas.

red clover

- Supports detoxification, relieves menopausal symptoms, and improves skin health.
- Typically brewed into teas or taken in supplement form.

rosemary

- Improves memory, relieves muscle pain, reduces inflammation and promotes hair growth.
- Used in cooking, as an essential oil for hair growth, or brewed into teas

sage

- Supports digestion, reduces inflammation, improves cognition.
- Used in cooking, brewed into teas, or taken in supplement form.

spearmint

- Aids digestion, relieves nausea, supports respiratory health.
- Often brewed into teas, used in culinary dishes, or taken in supplement form.

turmeric

- Anti-inflammatory, antioxidant, supports joint health.
- Used in cooking, brewed into teas, or taken in supplement form.

valerian

- Promotes relaxation, aids sleep, reduces anxiety.
- Typically brewed into teas or taken in supplement form as capsules or tinctures.

Each of these herbs carries a deep historical significance in medicine and provides many advantages for different health conditions. You can integrate them into your herbal arsenal according to your needs and preferences. It is essential to prioritize consulting a healthcare expert before starting a new herbal regimen, particularly if you have pre-existing medical conditions or are currently taking any medications despite the potential benefits associated with these herbs.

Practical Tips for Cultivating a Diverse Herbal Garden

Now that we have some ideas of the types of herbs available and their healing properties let's delve into practical tips that will help you cultivate a diverse herbal garden that reflects your unique style.

1. **Planning Your Garden:** Choose the herbs you'd like to see in your garden and use them. Think of their properties, how they may benefit you, and the colors and scents you want to see and smell. Do you constantly struggle with anxiety? Plant some lemon balm for teas. Lavender is perfect for crafting oils to gift to friends or family. Choose your plants according to your life and preferences, and don't be afraid to experiment with something new.

2. **Picking Your Space:** Your herbal garden can be as big or small as you prefer; only ensure sufficient room and sunlight in your location. Whether using a pre-made pot or building one yourself, it helps to learn about the herbs you plant. Knowing their growth patterns and recommended spacing requirements will ensure they can grow and thrive. Watch the space throughout the day and record the number of sunlight hours; plants require varying amounts of daily sunlight. Ensure your space has proper drainage; standing water can attract unwanted pests, and if you are high up, ensure you won't cause any damage below.

3. **Watering and Harvesting:** Like sunlight, plants require varying amounts of water. Try grouping and placing your plants based on this fact. It helps to have multiple beds or pots, but thorough planning can do the trick just as well.

Ensure you have sufficient tools for harvesting and study the proper methods for your garden.

Personal Narratives: Success Stories From Individuals Who Have Created Their Healing Gardens

The story of "The Floating Gardens of Kolkata" is a powerful and compelling testament to the transformative impact of gardening on lives, with a particular emphasis on its empowering effect on women in marginalized communities (Robert Chiocca, 2023). These distinctive floating gardens, or bheris, stand as beacons of empowerment for Kolkata's women, offering them more than just a means to financial independence. Engaging in cultivating and managing these gardens has equipped them with a sense of ownership and pride, significantly enhancing their self-esteem and the overall well-being of their community. Moreover, their involvement has fostered a strong sense of unity and mutual support among them, further amplifying the gardens' role as a catalyst for social change. This remarkable success story highlights the healing and transformative powers of gardening. It underscores its potential as a tool for socio-economic upliftment and community development, showcasing how it can positively change individual lives and broader communities.

THE SYMBIOSIS OF PLANTS AND MIND

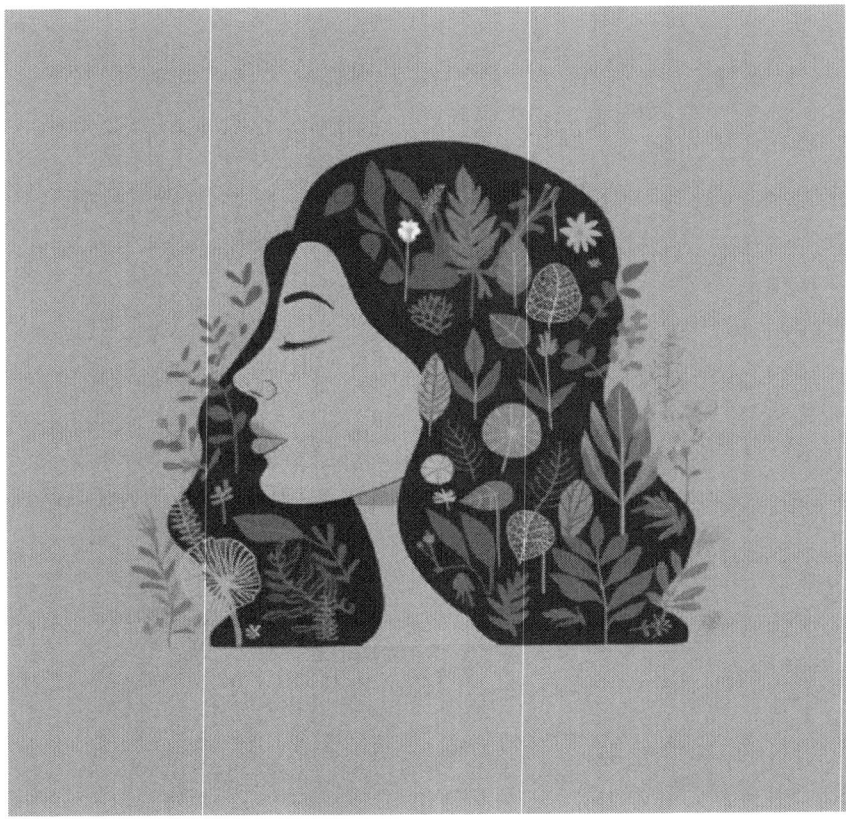

The human mind is a unique and intricate ecosystem comprising different sections, each with its purpose contributing to overall well-being. Our gardens should reflect this diversity if we hope to enjoy the full range of therapeutic benefits gardening offers. What if I told you that the vibrant colors of plants have been proven to stimulate the brain, boosting your creative motivation, or that merely having a plant nearby can enhance your concentration and memory?

Plants have a natural way of increasing happiness hormones and uplifting our moods by purely being in our presence. This may seem unsurprising, considering that our very survival relies on the resilience and endurance of plants. Everything from the air we breathe to the vegetables we eat or force our children to eat are products of our innate connection with nature and our brains. Perhaps our natural bond with nature uplifts our spirits whenever they are near.

The science backing the profound effects of plants and gardening on one's mental and physical well-being continues to grow. Studies have shown that exposure to nature and greenery, engaging in gardening activities, and even taking care of a simple house plant can reduce symptoms of depression, anxiety, and mood disorders.

Gardening is a powerful therapeutic tool that addresses mental health and psychological, spiritual, physical, and social needs. Let's talk about some natural benefits of gardening on the mind. Science has shown that exposure to soil and sunlight triggers the release of neurotransmitters that reduce anxiety and depression. They've found links to certain bacterium strains within the soil that aid in releasing serotonin, a mood-stabilizing hormone that fosters feelings of happiness. Sunlight exposure has proven an effective treatment for seasonal affective disorder (SAD), a type of depression associated with changes in seasons. Research has shown that gardening can serve as a helpful activity for dementia patients, allowing them to reminisce and engage in memory-sharing. These are just a few positive effects gardening can have on mental health.

Meditation and Mindfulness in the Herbal Garden

A thriving home garden can provide solace from the day's stresses, a serene escape perfect for practices in mindfulness and meditation. Mindfulness is an awareness of your emotions, mind, and body in the present moment. Practicing mindfulness incorporates techniques such as deep breathing, visualization, and other relaxation practices to calm the body and mind, ultimately easing stress. Through meditation, individuals learn to focus their attention and fully immerse themselves in the present moment, fostering a state of mindfulness. Like gardening, these practices have proven effective in reducing stress, promoting mental well-being, and enhancing overall health. Specifically, these activities can provide relief from symptoms of depression and anxiety.

With its calming environment, an herbal garden offers the perfect setting for visitors to release their worries and find tranquility, making it an ideal place for meditation. In a garden, one can truly connect with the living environment, promoting self-awareness and a sense of calm. Inhaling the aromatic scents of lavender, rosemary, and mint during meditation promotes a sense of tranquility and helps to foster a deeper state of relaxation and mindfulness.

If your garden space is too limited for meditation, fear not; you can still gain the mindful benefits of a garden environment. Simply being in the presence of your plants or keeping them in view can create a peaceful atmosphere.

Case Study: How a Mindful Herbal Garden Transformed One Person's Mental Health

Faris's journey in the world of gardening paints a vivid picture of the therapeutic impact of tending to plants on mental health, particularly for individuals grappling with conditions like depression and PTSD. His experience began when he received houseplants as a gift in his new apartment. The responsibility of caring for his plants, especially his mini bonsai tree, became a pivotal moment in his mental health journey. Faris encountered a challenging period where he neglected his bonsai, leading to its apparent demise. When he recommenced care, the guilt and subsequent revival of the plant symbolized hope and resilience. This singular bright green leaf that sprouted on the bonsai became a metaphor for his recovery and resurgence.

Faris's story underscores the psychological benefits of gardening, which align with research findings on the therapeutic effects of horticulture. Nurturing a living entity provides a sense of purpose and accomplishment, both critical factors in improving mental well-being. Moreover, observing growth and change in plants can be deeply rewarding and grounding.

For Faris, his indoor garden became a sanctuary, a place of refuge, where he could nurture life and find a reason to persevere through his darkest moments. Caring for plants and observing their growth can serve as a therapeutic routine for those with PTSD and depression. Gardening empowered him with a sense of control and responsibility, both of which are vital in managing mental health conditions.

This connection with nature, even in an urban setting, is crucial for mental health, offering an escape from the pressures and stimuli of daily life. Faris's experience is a testament to the healing power of gardening, demonstrating how it can transform mental health struggles into stories of resilience and hope. Crossley (2022) emphasizes the significance of finding joy and purpose in everyday activities and their profound effect on our mental and emotional well-being.

CHAPTER 2

Soil, Seeds, and Self-Care

Did you know that individuals who engage in gardening daily experience a notable enhancement in their well-being? A study has revealed that these avid gardeners have well-being scores that are 6.6% higher and stress levels that are 4.2% lower compared to those who do not partake in gardening (Sky News, 2021). We've discussed a few of the benefits of gardening on mental health and the science that backs it. This chapter will teach you more about caring for your herbal garden. We'll discuss soil care and gardening rituals for self-care. We'll talk more in-depth about selecting herbs for therapeutic goals and provide some tips for beginners on seed selection. Finally, we'll discuss incorporating herbs into your daily routines and review herbal teas, infusions, and their health benefits.

NURTURING THE SOIL, NURTURING THE SOUL

Your plants' health and the success of your herbal garden depend on the condition of your soil. Knowing some background on your plants, precisely the kinds of soil and drainage conditions they thrive in, is vital in the planning stages of your garden. It may seem daunting initially, but soil health is relatively simple and easy to maintain. With a few simple tips and tools, you'll become an expert in your plants and the soil they call home, how to test it, and the signs of when to change or fertilize it.

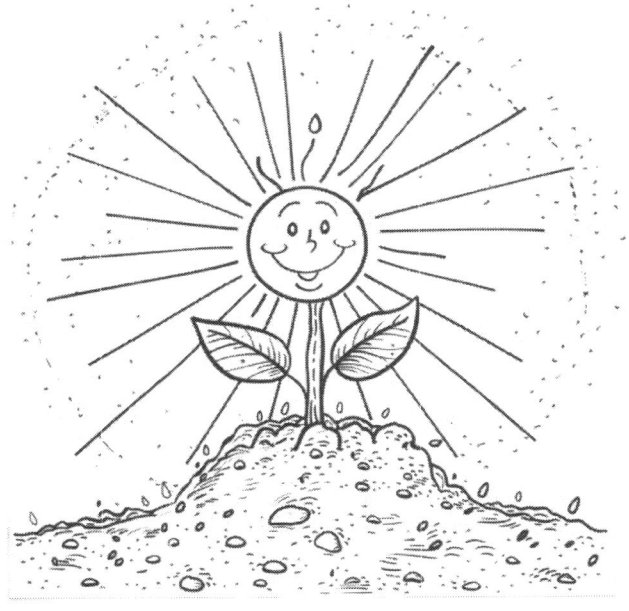

Like hours of sunlight and ounces of water, plants thrive in specific soil conditions. Plants rely on soil for nutrients, water intake, structure, and protection. We must know the specifics of these requirements to keep our plants healthy and robust. Here are a few general tips to remember when selecting soil for your garden and maintaining your soil health in the future.

When choosing soil for your herb garden, you can opt for store-bought brands, often specially crafted to fit the needs of certain plants, or you can try your hand at creating your custom mixes combined with the perfect blend of nutrients and minerals for your unique garden. Here are a few things to look for when choosing your soil, whether buying or crafting.

You'll want to choose soil that is well-draining. Herbs thrive best when planted in consistently damp soil, allowing the roots to absorb water. Consider mixtures of vermiculite or perlite if crafting them yourself, and if you have the space and time, consider mulching. Mulching is a process that converts dead leaves and other organic materials into a natural fertilizer, which is perfect for nourishing your garden. If you're in the market for soil mixes, prioritize organic ones packed with nutrients and slow-release fertilizers. You'll also want to monitor the pH levels in your soil. Most plants favor a range between six and seven. There are plenty of options if you're looking for an inexpensive soil pH tester. Adjusting the pH levels in your soil is possible through introducing various solvents. Remembering these tips will guide you in selecting and maintaining the optimal soil for your herbs, resulting in improved well-being for your garden and you.

If you want to be more actively involved, consider creating your mixture. Here are some tips to help you get started. First, you must decide on the soil blend you want for your herbs. Common soil types include loam, clay, sandy, silty, chalk, and peat. Each type is suitable for different plants and uses. You can also blend amendments into your soil to alter its structure. Let's discuss these soil types, possible amendments, and their best-suited plants and uses.

These Are the Common Soils:

- Loam soil is a popular choice for many gardeners, as it combines sand, silt, and clay. It resembles clay soil but provides better drainage while retaining enough moisture for plant roots. It's used for planting various herbs, including basil, thyme, and rosemary.

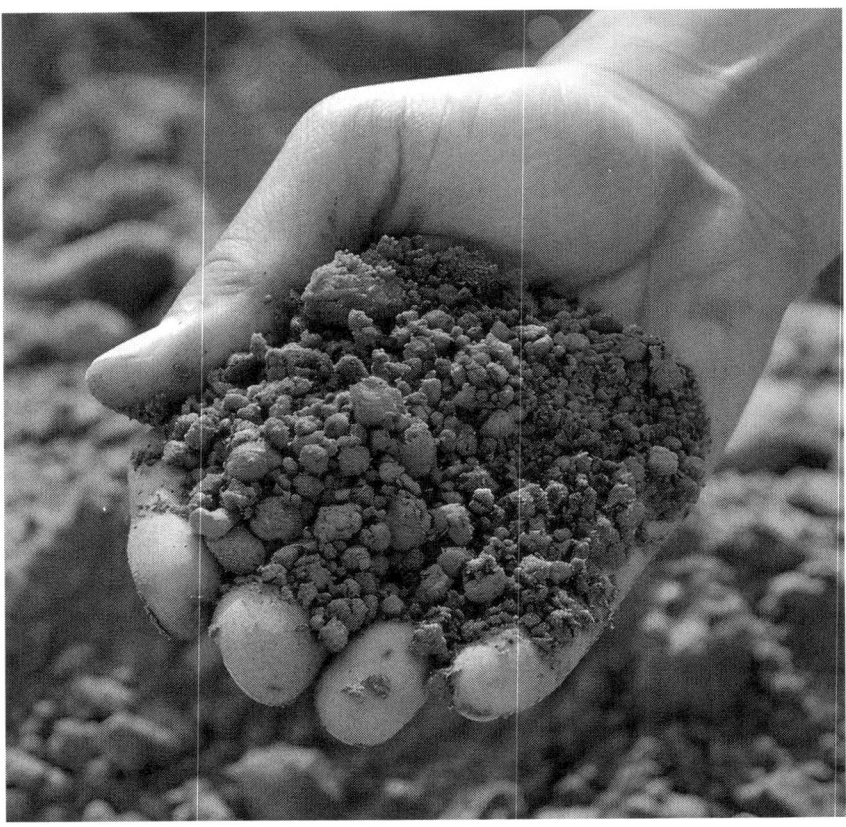

- Clay soil is heavy and tends to become compacted. It retains water well but can become waterlogged, leading to poor drainage. Herbs that can tolerate clay soil include mint, chives, and lavender.

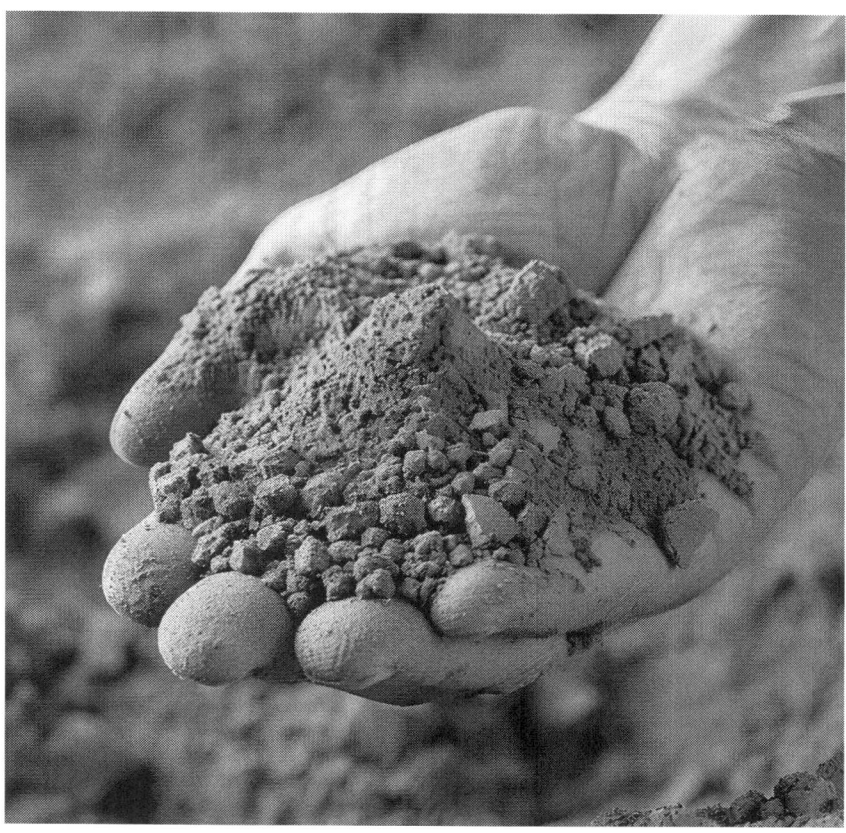

- Sandy soil looks grainy, is well-draining, and does not easily retain water or nutrients. It is best suited for drought-tolerant herbs such as sage, oregano, and marjoram.

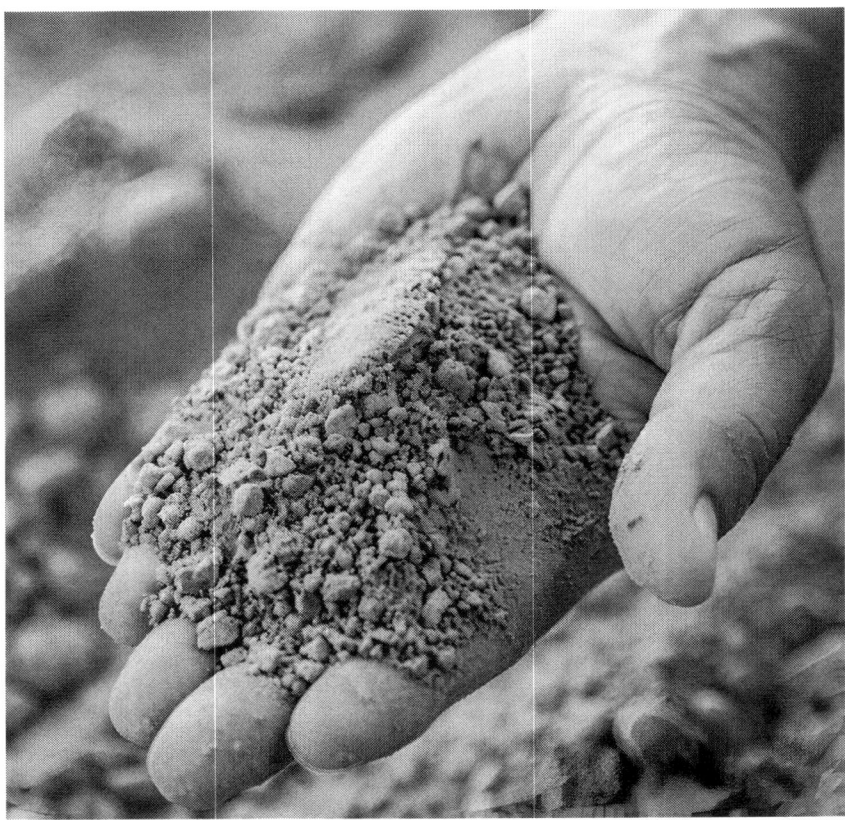

- Silty soil is smooth and fine-textured, retaining moisture but draining well. It is suitable for herbs like parsley, cilantro, and dill.

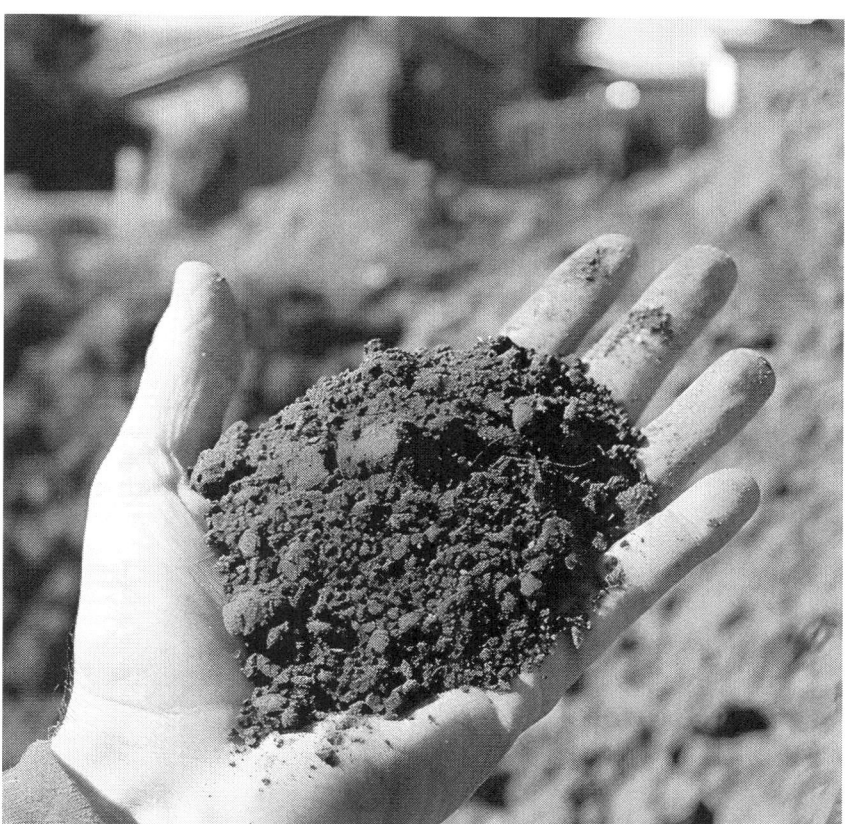

- Chalky soil is alkaline and often lacks essential nutrients. Herbs that thrive in chalky soil include thyme, lavender, and rosemary.

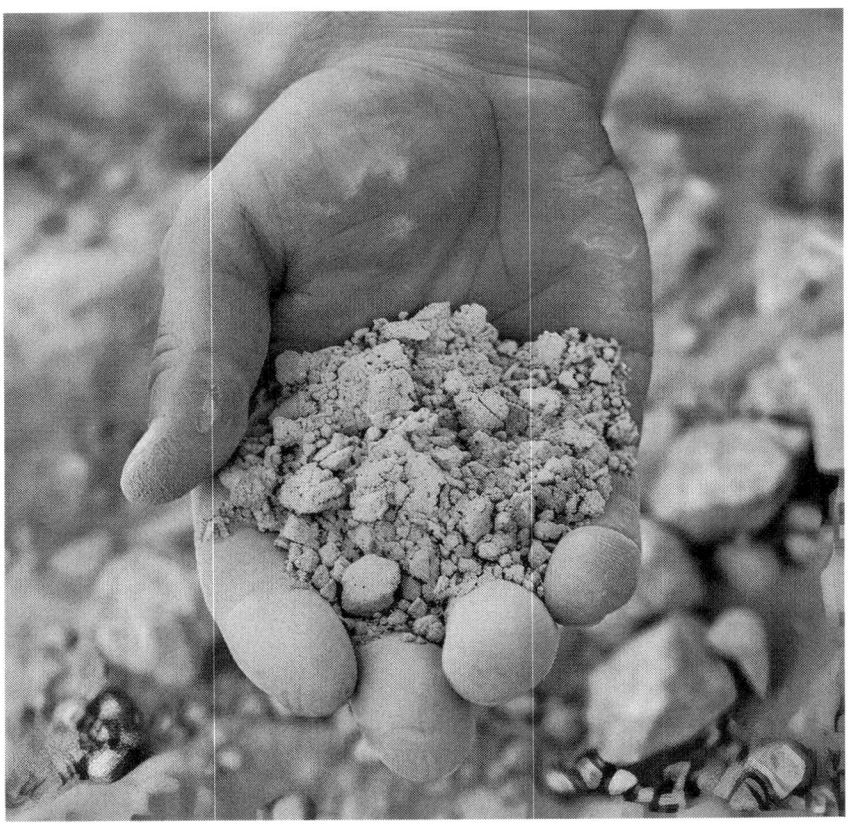

- Peat soil is acidic and retains moisture well. It is commonly used for growing herbs such as mint, lemon balm, and coriander.

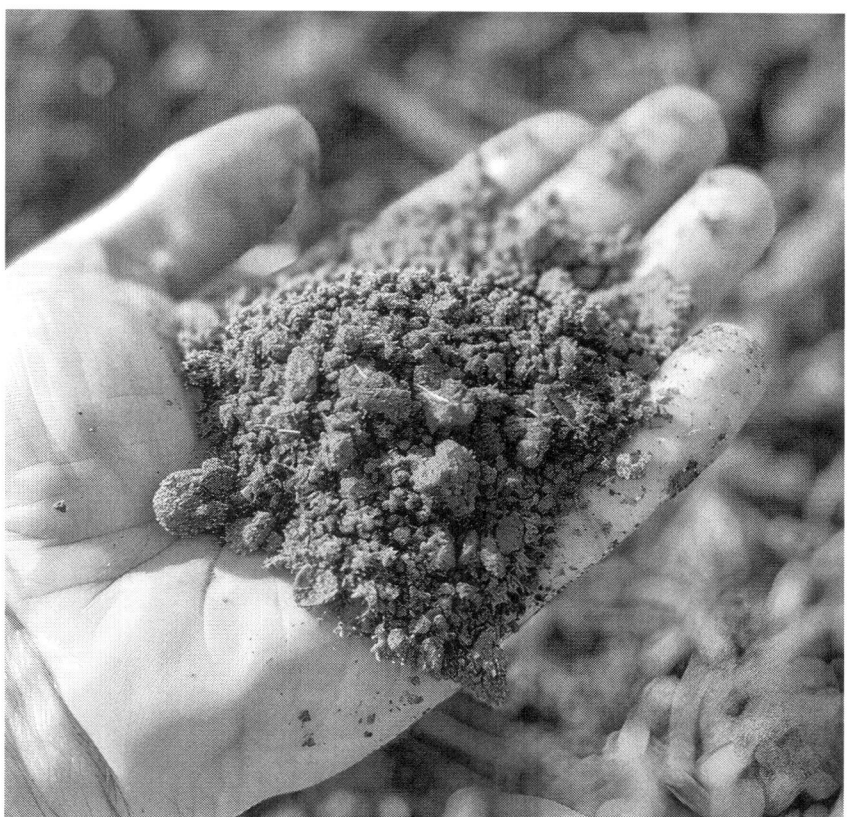

Amendments

Soil amendments are like the condiments of your soil; they're materials mixed into the soil to enhance properties such as drainage, aeration, retention, and fertility. Some of the more common types used in soil for herbs include compost, peat moss, vermiculite, perlite, and sand. Compost is rich in organic matter and adds nutrients to the soil, improving its fertility. Peat moss helps retain moisture and improve drainage. Vermiculite and perlite are lightweight materials that will enhance soil aeration and drainage. You can add sand to heavy clay soils to improve drainage.

You can mix these soil amendments in different quantities depending on the needs of your plants. These additions can improve the overall health and productivity of the soil, providing a favorable environment for herbs to thrive. When crafting soil for herbal gardening, understanding the properties and uses of various soil amendments is crucial. Let's explore coconut coir, peat moss, compost, perlite, and topsoil:

1. **Coconut Coir:** Made from the fiber of coconut husks, coconut coir is an excellent soil amendment. It improves soil aeration and retains moisture effectively. It's often used in hydroponic systems and is a sustainable alternative to peat moss.

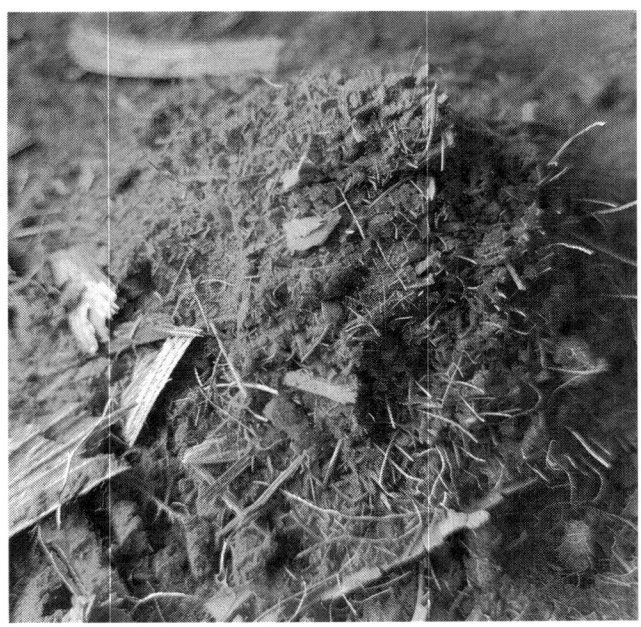

2. Peat Moss: Peat moss, sourced from decomposed plant material in peat bogs, has a distinct acidic scent. Peat moss is acidic and has a high capacity for water retention. It's commonly used to improve soil texture and moisture holding in gardens.

3. Compost: Compost, rich in organic matter, is crucial for improving soil fertility and structure. It adds essential nutrients, improves drainage and water retention, and is beneficial for almost all types of gardening, including herbal gardens.

4. Perlite: This volcanic glass expands into a lightweight, porous material when heated. Perlite enhances soil drainage and aeration, making it ideal for preventing soil compaction, particularly in container gardening.

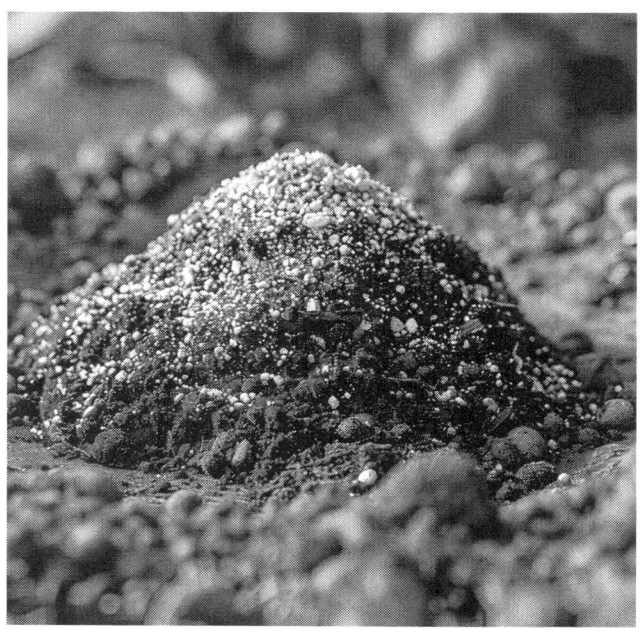

5. Topsoil: The uppermost layer of soil, topsoil, is rich in organic matter and nutrients. Gardeners use topsoil as the primary medium for planting and often enrich it with other amendments to cater to specific gardening needs, such as herbal gardening.

The right combinations of these components can create an optimal growing environment for herbs, balancing moisture retention, aeration, and nutrient supply.

Once you have decided on the types of soil and amendments that suit your herbs, you can start making your mix by combining these soils in the desired ratios. Keep track of moisture levels and adjust your watering routine accordingly. When starting your garden with this hands-on approach, you can craft a unique blend of soil that will help your herbs thrive. If you need help deciding on the soil mixture for your herbal garden, below are a few suggestions to guide you.

Our Recommendations for Your Herbal Garden Soil Mix

As stated, we recommend a well-draining soil mixture for your herbal garden. Combining garden soil, compost, perlite, or vermiculite can balance nutrients and moisture retention. Organic materials such as compost can enhance soil fertility and promote the healthy growth of your herbs. Testing the soil's pH level and making necessary adjustments is also advisable, as most herbs prefer a slightly acidic to neutral pH. Lastly, consider the specific requirements of the herbs you plan to grow and tailor the soil mixture accordingly. For example, herbs like lavender and rosemary thrive in sandy, well-draining soil, while mint and basil prefer slightly moist soil. It may take some research to get the right soil blend, but countless resources are available; keep this guide handy, and don't be afraid to experiment.

From the website Housegrail, Peter Ortiz suggests using a mixture of equal parts coconut coir or peat moss, compost, perlite, and topsoil for growing herbs (Ortiz, 2023). This mixture can be used as a starting point, and you can make adjustments in the future as needed.

Below is my step-by-step process for preparing your soil for maximum results:

Step 1: Collecting Soil Samples

- Choose several locations within your garden area to collect soil samples. For each location, dig a hole 6-8 inches deep and take a small scoop of soil from the bottom of the hole.
- Combine the samples from different locations into one clean container to get a composite sample representing your garden area.
- Allow the soil to dry at room temperature, removing any stones, roots, or debris.

Step 2: Testing for Nutrient Levels and pH

- You can use a home soil test kit at garden centers or online. These kits usually include tools and instructions for testing pH, nitrogen (N), phosphorus (P), and potassium (K) levels.
- Follow the kit's instructions carefully. Typically, this involves mixing your soil sample with water and a test chemical and then comparing the color change to a chart provided.

- For a more comprehensive analysis, consider sending your soil sample to a local extension service or soil testing laboratory. They can provide detailed insights into your soil's condition, including micronutrient levels and specific recommendations for amendments.

Step 3: Interpreting Results and Planning Amendments

- The pH scale ranges from 0 to 14, with seven being neutral. Most herbs prefer a slightly acidic to neutral pH (6.0 to 7.0). If your soil is too acidic (pH below 6), you'll need to add lime. If it's too alkaline (pH above 7), sulfur will help lower the pH.
- Nutrient levels will be indicated as low, medium, or high. Based on your results, you'll identify which nutrients are lacking and must be supplemented.

Amending Soil

Inorganic Amendments

- Lime (calcium carbonate) increases soil pH, making it less acidic. Apply lime according to the test recommendations and your garden size.
- Sulfur lowers soil pH, making it more acidic. Use elemental sulfur as directed for your specific soil type and pH goal.
- Balanced NPK fertilizers or specific nutrient amendments like bone meal (for phosphorus) or greensand (for potassium) can address nutrient deficiencies. Use according to package instructions based on your soil test results.

Organic Matter Incorporation

Step 1: Choosing Organic Matter

- Compost: Decomposed organic material that enriches the soil with nutrients and beneficial microorganisms.
- Manure: Animal waste that provides a rich nutrient source. Use well-composted manure to avoid pathogens and weed seeds.
- Leaf Mold: Decomposed leaves that improve soil structure and water retention.

Step 2: Application

- Spread a 2-4-inch layer of organic matter over your garden area.
- Use a garden fork or tiller to incorporate the organic matter into the top 6-8 inches of soil. This enhances the soil structure, making it more friable and improving root penetration.

Step 3: Mulching

- After planting, apply a layer of organic mulch (straw, wood chips, or leaf mold) around your plants. This helps retain soil moisture, suppress weeds, and gradually adds organic matter to the soil as it decomposes.

Final Steps

- Water the area thoroughly after amending to help integrate the amendments and organic matter into the soil.
- Allow the soil to settle for a few days before planting your herbs.

By carefully testing and amending your soil and incorporating rich organic matter, you create a fertile and sustainable environment that will nurture your herbal garden for future seasons.

Gardening Rituals for Self-Care

You've likely heard of self-care rituals. These routine activities are meant to replenish the mind, body, and soul. Herbal gardening provides a unique self-care experience, offering a tranquil connection with nature and the soothing benefits of exotic scents, vibrant colors, and health-restoring herbs. In this section, we'll explore a few self-care rituals for gardening and how they can benefit you.

1. **Mindful Weeding and Planting:** This ritual focuses entirely on the task and your senses as you do it. Experience the soft textures of the soil while digging your hands into the earth. Gaze on the vibrant colors of the plants and leaves throughout your garden. You can reduce stress and anxiety by grounding and centering your thoughts through this practice.
2. **Crafting Homemade Herbal Teas:** Experience the satisfaction of harvesting your herbs, such as mint, chamomile, or lemon balm, and transforming them into comforting herbal teas that fill your space with delightful

scents. Carefully selecting, cleaning, and steeping the herbs can create a soothing and fulfilling experience, instilling a sense of achievement.

3. **Garden Journaling:** In a dedicated journal, capture your gardening journey's sights, sounds, and progress. Note the vibrant plant growth, create a visual representation of your garden layout, or express your innermost thoughts and feelings. Journaling in your garden allows for a reflective experience, enhancing mindfulness.

4. **Sunrise or Sunset Gardening:** Align your gardening with the sunrise or sunset. This timing offers the perfect lighting conditions for gardening and imbues the surroundings with tranquility, taking the experience to a spiritual plane.

Making these exercises part of your routine may require some dedication. But as you witness the growth and blossoming of your garden, you may discover a similar development within yourself. Maintaining your garden with commitment and perseverance transforms it into a rewarding and engaging practice. Remember to experiment with different activities that may benefit you specifically. By making this self-care habit a regular part of your life, you can experience lasting improvements in your mental, physical, and emotional health.

Anecdote: A Personal Journey of Healing Through Soil Connection

The concept of healing through soil connection is impactful and encompasses the transformative journey of both the land and the individual. At the Garden of L.E.A.H., one practice that highlights the symbiotic relationship between humans and the earth is using green manure by turning weeds. As the soil becomes more biodiverse, it begins to heal, and a parallel personal healing process occurs. By accepting the natural cycle of life and grasping the interconnectedness of all beings, individuals can attain profound mindfulness and self-awareness. This journey is not just about the physical labor of working with the soil but encompasses the mental and emotional well-being fostered by this connection. Scientific findings show that soil bacteria can positively impact human health (Breeshop, 2019).

CHOOSING AND PLANTING SEEDS WITH INTENT

When exploring the vast and engaging world of plants and herbs, it's essential to approach the selection of herbs for your garden with intent. Throughout this journey, we have emphasized the importance of designing a garden that truly embodies who you are. Its location, dimensions, and the plants it supports should all align with your unique needs and desires. Let's review a few tips for selecting seeds for your herbal garden.

Let's delve into the plant's therapeutic attributes and medicinal advantages. Select plants that will aid you in your garden by how they will benefit your body and mind. Create a list of the common issues you experience, including headaches, depression, skin irritations, and similar ailments. Cross-reference these with plants known for their medicinal properties that may assist with these ailments. Remember to check out our section from Chapter 1, titled *Essential Herbs for Therapeutic Gardening*, if you need any help.

It's essential to consider the aesthetics, including the visual appeal and overall atmosphere. Consider choosing plants with scents that you find appealing or colors that create a striking contrast with their surroundings. Consider your taste preferences and choose herbs that complement the flavors you enjoy or use frequently in your cooking. If you plan a specific diet, select herbs to help you achieve your goals, such as incorporating more greens into your meals for healthier eating or using peppermint to relieve muscle soreness after intense workouts. Consider adding some echinacea to your garden to prepare for the cold season. Your herbal garden holds infinite potential, with endless options and combinations to choose from.

We must also consider the environmental elements that may affect your garden. Research which plants thrive in your climate, as temperature can significantly impact their health. Ensure plenty of room for your plants to spread out and flourish. Remember the height and sunlight preferences of the herbs you decide on, and consider what materials you have.

Consider your plants' care and maintenance requirements when planning your herbal garden. Carefully consider the specific fertilizer they need and the quantity of water they require. By keeping these factors in mind, you can ensure that you select the perfect plants and seeds for your garden, creating an aromatic and visually appealing oasis.

Seed Starting Guide for Beginners

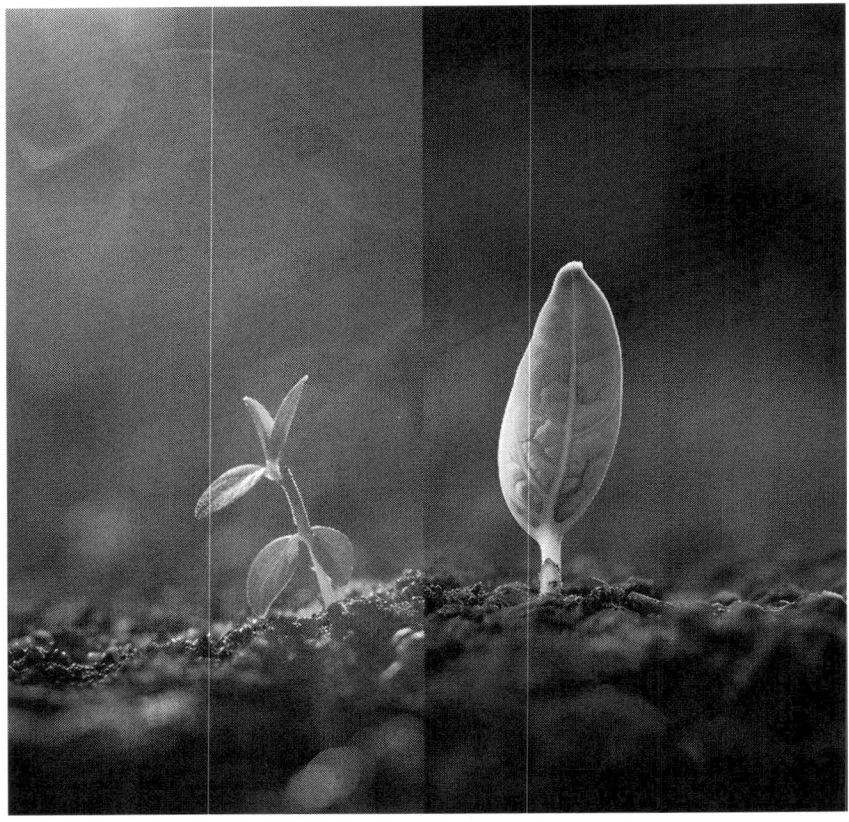

Although planting pre-sprouted herbs is a time-saver, starting from seeds is a rewarding experience. By starting with seeds, gardeners can witness the complete growth cycle of plants, nurturing, watering, and pruning them throughout the process. This cycle provides a fascinating glimpse into the growth habits of herbs, equipping you with valuable knowledge for your future gardening pursuits.

When selecting seeds, opt for high-quality ones to achieve optimal results. Remember, knowing the precise soil, temperature, and light preferences of the herb you intend to cultivate is essential for success. In the next section, we'll break down the process of starting seeds in your herbal garden into easy-to-follow steps.

1. **Soil Preparation:** Carefully select a sterile, well-draining seed starting mix. Avoid using garden soil, as it may harbor pathogens detrimental to delicate seedlings.
2. **Sowing Seeds:** Gently plant the seeds at the precise depth of the seed packet, carefully following the instructions. Scatter delicate seeds that crave sunlight on the soil surface, allowing their potential to bloom under the radiant rays. On the other hand, certain seeds demand a tender covering of soil, as if tucked into a cozy bed, ready to nurture their growth.
3. **Watering:** Gently moisten the soil to avoid waterlogging. The delicate sound of droplets from a spray bottle fills the air, preventing the risk of overwatering. This method ensures that tiny seeds remain undisturbed.
4. **Providing Light:** Place the seed trays in a brightly illuminated space to ensure optimal growth, allowing the vibrant rays to cascade upon the delicate herbs. Alternatively, harness the radiance of grow lights, casting a warm and nurturing glow upon the seeds. These light sources serve as a beacon, beckoning the herbs to sprout and flourish, giving them vitality.
5. **Temperature Control:** Ensure a steady, optimal environment that caters to the unique needs of your herb seeds. Immerse yourself in a world where warmth permeates the air, creating a cozy haven for germination. With each breath, the gentle hum of the temperature

regulator soothes your senses, blending seamlessly with the faint aroma of earth and anticipation.

6. **Thinning Seedlings:** As the seedlings sprout their delicate first true leaves, gently pluck out the excess to avoid overcrowding. This allows the vibrant plants to bask in ample space for their growth, creating a harmonious sight of thriving greenery. The soft rustle of leaves and the subtle scent of fresh earth fill the air, providing a tranquil ambiance. By thinning the seedlings, you ensure the best chance for robust growth, delighting in the tactile sensation of nurturing life.

Case Study: Overcoming Challenges in the Early Stages of Herbal Gardening

Transitioning from indoor to outdoor community gardening can be a challenging learning experience, especially for those new to herbal gardening. One gardener's story of moving herbs like rosemary, lavender, and cilantro from indoors to the community garden is relatable for many first-time gardeners. Unfortunately, the herbs withered unexpectedly, teaching the gardener the importance of understanding local growing seasons and environmental conditions like frost. This narrative highlights the need for patience and learning from experience when cultivating a successful garden. It serves as a case study in adapting to the challenges of early-stage gardening (Curtis, 2023).

DAILY PRACTICES FOR HERBAL SELF-CARE

With our seeds planted and our eyes on the soil, waiting for that first sprout, let's explore ways we can use these herbs daily. Blending your herbs into daily self-care routines can be as beneficial as gardening. Herbs provide a flavor and fragrance to our foods while also providing health benefits. They can relieve stress and pain through aroma baths and herbal ointments. Here are some ways we can maximize the use of these herbs in our everyday lives:

1. **Herbal Infusions:** Chamomile for relaxation, peppermint for digestion, or lavender for stress relief can provide a soothing and rejuvenating effect.
2. **Aromatherapy:** Harness the power of essential oils derived from herbs to create a calming and uplifting atmosphere. Adding a few drops of your favorite herbal oil to your diffuser or bathwater will promote relaxation and relieve stress.
3. **DIY Herbal Skincare:** Many herbs possess properties that can benefit our skin. You can create herbal skincare products by infusing herbs into oils or using them in homemade face masks and scrubs. Calendula, rosemary, and aloe vera are some herbs that can nourish and rejuvenate your skin.
4. **Culinary Adventures:** Experiment with incorporating fresh herbs into your cooking. Not only do they add flavor and aroma to your dishes, but they also provide essential nutrients. Basil, cilantro, thyme, and parsley are popular herbs among chefs worldwide.
5. **Herbal Baths:** Treat yourself to a relaxing herbal bath. Tie a bunch of fresh herbs like rosemary or lavender

together and toss them into a warm bath. The aromatic steam will create a spa-like experience, while the herbs can help soothe muscles and promote relaxation.

Incorporate herbs into your daily self-care routines and experiment with different varieties to find what works best for your day and health. Enjoy nurturing your herbs and reaping the rewards they bring to your overall well-being.

Personal Anecdotes: Daily Rituals That Have Brought Tranquility to Real Lives

Mark's experience in Los Angeles is an excellent example of how incorporating daily rituals such as sunset yoga by the ocean can significantly improve one's tranquility and mental clarity. His daily routine of practicing yoga with the gentle waves and warm sand of the sea as a backdrop shows how connecting with nature can bring peace and rejuvenate the mind. This practice helped him relax and gave him the energy and calmness needed to handle his demanding role as an executive more effectively (Singh, 2023).

CHAPTER 3
Seasons of Healing

Have you ever considered how a garden mirrors the cycles of healing and growth in our lives in its ever-changing seasonal glory? Just as a garden evolves through the seasons, from the dormant quiet of winter to the vibrant bloom of spring, our journeys of healing and rejuvenation are reflected in the evolution of our minds and bodies.

The life cycle of herbs is an intricate and fascinating process that unfolds gradually as the seasons change. Each season brings a unique set of environmental conditions that shape the growth and development of the herb. From the first buds that emerge in spring to the seed production in fall, the life cycle of the herb is marked by distinct stages characterized by changes in its appearance, aroma, and taste.

In spring, the herb starts its life cycle with the emergence of tender buds that gradually grow into lush green leaves. As the days get warmer and longer, the herb enters a rapid growth and development phase, producing new shoots and branches. In summer, the herb reaches its peak growth and delivers beautiful flowers that attract bees and other pollinators. The flowers are visually pleasing and are crucial to the herb's reproductive cycle.

As summer ends, the herb produces seeds for its next life cycle. The seeds culminate in the herb's growth and development and contain all the genetic information necessary for the next generation of herbs. In fall, the seeds are mature and ready to be harvested, and the herb starts to wither and die, preparing for the winter months ahead.

In conclusion, the life cycle of herbs is a complex and intricate process that unfolds gradually over the changing seasons. Each herb's life cycle stage is marked by unique characteristics reflecting seasonal changes and environmental conditions.

SPRING RENEWAL AND GROWTH

Spring brings nature to the forefront, and vibrant colors fill the air, creating the perfect backdrop for exploring the healing properties of different herbs. Next, we will provide a few recommendations for spring herbs. Several environmental factors contribute to the renewal and growth of plant life in spring.

As winter draws close, the days become longer, and the temperature rises. Increasing sunlight and warmth allows plants to start photosynthesizing and producing energy. The melting of snow and ice rehydrates the cold, hardened soil, allowing plants to access the water they need for growth. The changing weather patterns in spring often bring rainfall, which further supports plant growth by providing additional moisture and nutrients to the soil. This renewal and growth in spring are vital parts of the plant life cycle, ensuring the survival and reproduction of various plant species.

Herbs for Spring Healing

- **Lavender:** Lavender is a well-known herb often used for its calming scent. It is a popular choice for relaxation and stress relief. It's particularly effective in alleviating anxiety and promoting better sleep, making it a spring essential for a calm mind.
- **Chamomile:** This gentle herb, with its daisy-like flowers, is known for its digestive and soothing properties. Chamomile tea is perfect for soothing an upset stomach, aiding relaxation, and providing better sleep quality during restless spring nights.
- **Peppermint:** A revitalizing herb, peppermint is excellent for respiratory health. Its refreshing scent can help clear sinuses and relieve seasonal allergies expected in spring.
- **Echinacea:** With its immune-boosting properties, echinacea is ideal for preparing the body against late spring colds, enhancing overall immunity.
- **Calendula:** Known for its skin-healing properties, calendula is perfect for repairing winter-worn skin. It's used in creams and salves for its soothing effect on irritated or dry skin.
- **Lemon Balms:** This herb is a mood lifter, helping to alleviate springtime blues with its uplifting citrus scent, and is also beneficial in calming nerves and improving digestion.

Integrate these spring herbs into your daily routine to harness their benefits. Add fresh lavender to your pillow for better sleep, sip on chamomile tea for digestive ease, or use peppermint oil for respiratory relief. Plant these herbs in your garden or pots to enjoy their therapeutic presence daily.

GARDENING ACTIVITIES FOR THE SEASON

Spring gardening is a time of bustling activity and preparation. Start by preparing the soil for new growth; enrich it with compost or organic matter to ensure it's fertile and ready for planting. This season is ideal for sowing seeds of herbs and flowers and transplanting seedlings that were started indoors. Early spring is also the time to prune back any overwintered plants, encouraging fresh growth. Implement early pest control measures, such as introducing beneficial insects or natural deterrents, to protect young plants from common spring pests.

Spring offers a unique opportunity for mindfulness and personal growth. Engage with your garden as a task and as a serene retreat. Take the time to notice the new buds forming, the birds returning, and the gradual lengthening of the days. Activities like planting and pruning can become meditative, connecting you with the cycle of life and renewal. Enjoy the unfolding beauty and the tactile experience of working with the soil and plants. This mindful engagement can be a source of tranquility and a reminder of nature's resilience and perpetual renewal.

Case Study: A Spring Herbal Garden Transformation

In this case study, we'll talk about the story of a homeowner's efforts to turn their backyard into an exquisite and functional outdoor space. The project focused on creating a spring herb garden near the kitchen. Despite the budget, time constraints, and weather conditions, the project was completed in stages, emphasizing the importance of timing in planting. The herb garden became a practical addition for culinary purposes and a source of immense joy and satisfaction. The ability to easily access fresh herbs and the pleasure of viewing the garden from the kitchen window exemplified the personal fulfillment derived from this gardening project (Jami, 2019).

SUMMER ABUNDANCE AND ENERGY

The garden is a sight to behold during the summer months. As the sun shines down, the herbs in the garden seem to come alive, reaching their peak potency. The vibrant colors of the herbs create a stunning display, with shades of green, purple, and yellow painting a beautiful picture. The air is filled with a refreshing fragrance as the herbs release their aromatic oils into the surroundings. This pleasant scent invigorates the senses and uplifts the mood of anyone who walks through the garden. Not only are the herbs visually appealing and fragrant, but they also possess energizing properties. Their leaves are filled with essential oils and compounds that are physically and mentally revitalizing. The garden becomes a haven of vitality, where one can experience the power of nature's healing properties. Summertime herbs thrive in the summer sun, making them perfect for promoting health and wellness. Summer's herbs offer unique health benefits; here, we've listed a few.

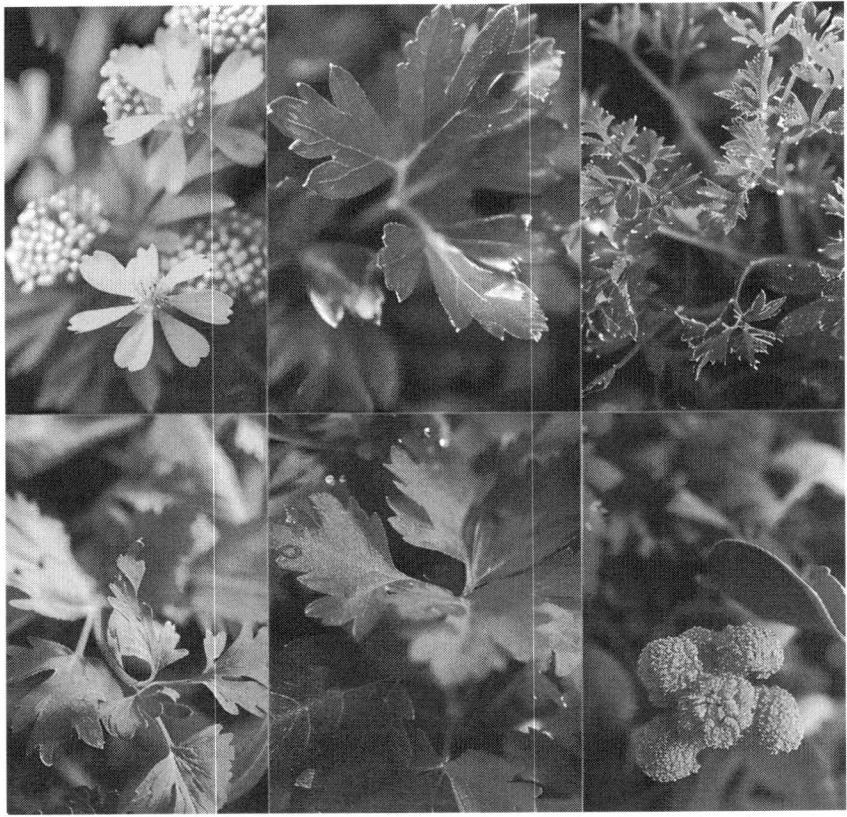

1. **St. John's Wort:** Many people choose St. John's Wort for its celebrated mood-enhancing properties, which help ease mild depression and anxiety.

2. **Lady's Bedstraw:** This plant is known for its detoxifying properties, which greatly aid in purifying the body.

3. **Cilantro:** Cilantro, bursting with antioxidants, supports detoxification and can help in heavy metal cleansing.

4. **Oregano:** Oregano offers an ideal way to boost the immune system and is well known for its anti-inflammatory effects because of its richness in antimicrobial properties.

5. **Parsley:** Parsley, a nutrient powerhouse, aids in digestion and supports kidney health.

Incorporating these herbs into your daily life is a breeze. For a calming experience, St. John's Wort and lavender can be infused in hot water to create a soothing tea or added to a diffuser as essential oils. Adding cilantro and parsley to your salads and dishes enhances the flavor and provides a nutritious boost. The scent of peppermint is refreshing, making it an ideal addition to herbal teas or a natural flavor for desserts.

Incorporating summer herbs into your daily routine is easy and fulfilling. You can use them in cooking to add nutrition and flavor, make herbal teas for health benefits, or create topical applications like salves or ointments. Each herb has a unique way of enhancing well-being, representing the energy and abundance of summer.

DIY Herbal Remedies for Common Ailments

Creating DIY herbal remedies can be both therapeutic and effective for various ailments. Here's a collection of recipes for teas, ointments, creams, and tinctures, complete with brief descriptions of each type of remedy:

Herbal Teas:

- **Peppermint Tea for Digestion:** To aid digestion and ease symptoms of irritable bowel syndrome, soak dried peppermint leaves in hot water for 7-10 minutes. Then, enjoy a soothing cup of peppermint tea.
- **Chamomile Tea for Relaxation:** Use dried chamomile

flowers steeped in hot water for a soothing, sleep-inducing drink.

Ointments and Creams:

- **Calendula Cream for Skin Healing:** Infuse calendula petals in a carrier oil, almond and olive are popular choices; strain and mix with beeswax to create a soothing cream for cuts and bruises.
- **Lavender Ointment for Stress Relief:** Blend lavender essential oil with a base ointment for a calming and relaxing topical application.

Tinctures:

- **Echinacea Tincture for Immune Support:** Soak echinacea root in alcohol for several weeks, strain, and use a few drops daily to boost the immune system.
- **St. John's Wort Tincture for Mood Enhancement:** Infuse dried St. John's Wort in alcohol to create a tincture that can help alleviate mild depression and anxiety.

Herbal Infused Oils:

- **Rosemary Hair Oil:** Rosemary hair oil is made by infusing rosemary in a carrier oil for several weeks. By using it, you can experience the growth of thick, beautiful hair and the revitalization of your scalp.
- **Oregano Infused Oil for Cooking:** Infuse dried oregano in olive oil to add a flavorful and healthy touch to your meals.

Each recipe offers a natural way to address common health concerns. When preparing these remedies, always use high-quality, organic ingredients. Start with small amounts to see how your body reacts. Remember, these natural remedies can complement but not replace medical advice from healthcare professionals.

Incorporate these DIY herbal remedies into your routine. Herbs' natural healing properties can enhance your daily self-care practices.

Anecdotes: How Summer Herbs Have Empowered Individuals to Take Control of Their Health

Linda B. White, M.D., from Golden, Colorado, shares her experience with lemon balm, highlighting its therapeutic and medicinal qualities. Among various mints, lemon balm stands out in her garden for its beauty and resilience. She notes its calming effects when consumed fresh and its utility in combating cold and flu symptoms when used in teas, tinctures, and syrups. This demonstrates how lemon balm has empowered her to take control of her health and well-being, utilizing the herb's antiviral, antibacterial, and other beneficial properties (Companion, 2001).

FALL HARVEST AND REFLECTION

Fall is known as the harvest season, a particular time of the year when many of your herbs and plants will finally become harvest-ready. During fall, the hard work and patience you put into cultivating your herbs and plants throughout the year will finally pay off. Nature showers us with a plentiful harvest during this season. The changing leaves, crisp air, and vibrant colors create a picturesque backdrop for this particular time of the year.

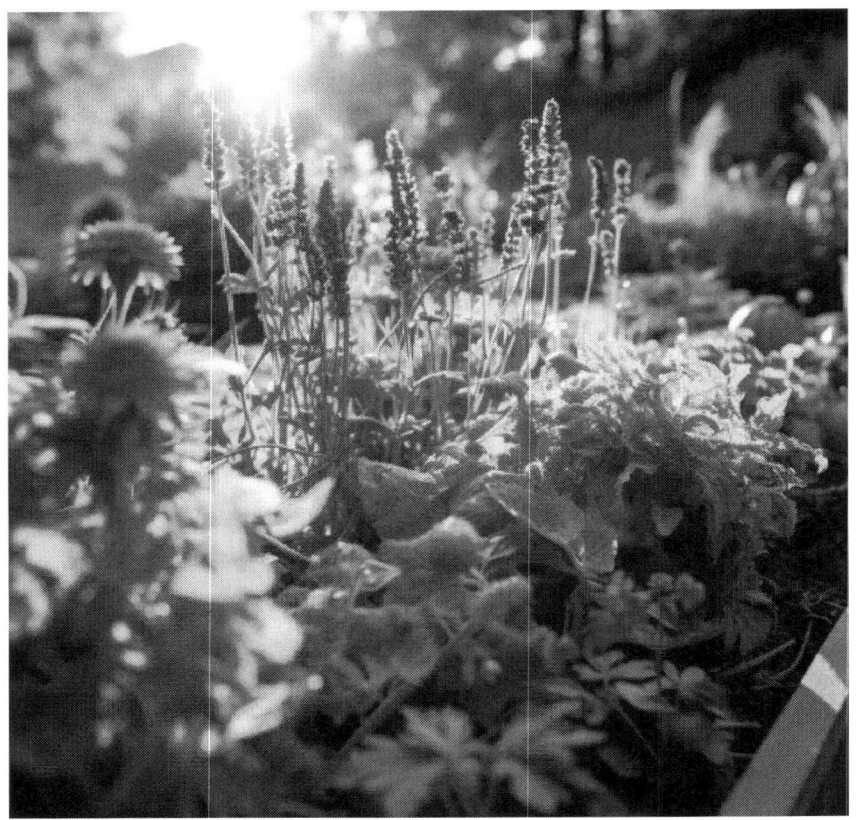

As the days grow shorter and the temperatures gradually drop, your garden becomes a treasure trove of ripe fruits, vegetables, and aromatic herbs. The once tender seedlings have matured into robust plants, ready to be plucked and enjoyed. Use the vibrant hues of purple basil, fragrant rosemary, and lush mint leaves to add a touch of freshness and aromatic splendor to your Thanksgiving cuisine.

Harvesting during this time requires careful observation and attention to detail. You must choose the perfect moment when the fruits and herbs peak ripeness, ensuring optimum flavor and nutritional value. With gentle hands, you pluck the fruits, gently separating them from their vines, taking care not to damage the delicate foliage. The satisfaction of gathering the fruits of your labor fills your heart with a sense of accomplishment and gratitude.

The harvest season is not just about reaping the rewards of your hard work but also a time to celebrate and share the abundance with others. You can gather with loved ones to prepare hearty meals using freshly harvested ingredients or preserve them for the colder months ahead. Preserve your fall harvest to enjoy seasonal flavors beyond autumn.

Preserving Herbs for Winter Use

You can preserve your harvest in various ways, depending on the herbs, fruits, or vegetables you grow. Herbs are likely the easiest to store. A simple mason jar, plastic zipper bag, Tupperware container, or plastic wrap can preserve your herbs for months. Check the specific conditions and expiration times for your freshly picked herbs. Infusing your herbs allows you to create delicious pastes, sauces, or oils that can be enjoyed on toast or used as toppings for desserts and salads. Additionally, you can make homemade sauces, such as tomato sauce or salsa, using your freshly harvested tomatoes, peppers, and herbs. These preserved goods provide sustenance during winter and make thoughtful gifts for friends and neighbors.

Moreover, sharing your abundance with others can foster community and gratitude as you celebrate the bountiful harvest and the joy of giving. Whether through a potluck dinner or donating excess produce to local food banks, sharing ensures everyone can enjoy the harvest's abundance. So, as the season transitions and the air turns chilly, take the time to preserve and share the flavors of fall, spreading warmth and cheer throughout your community.

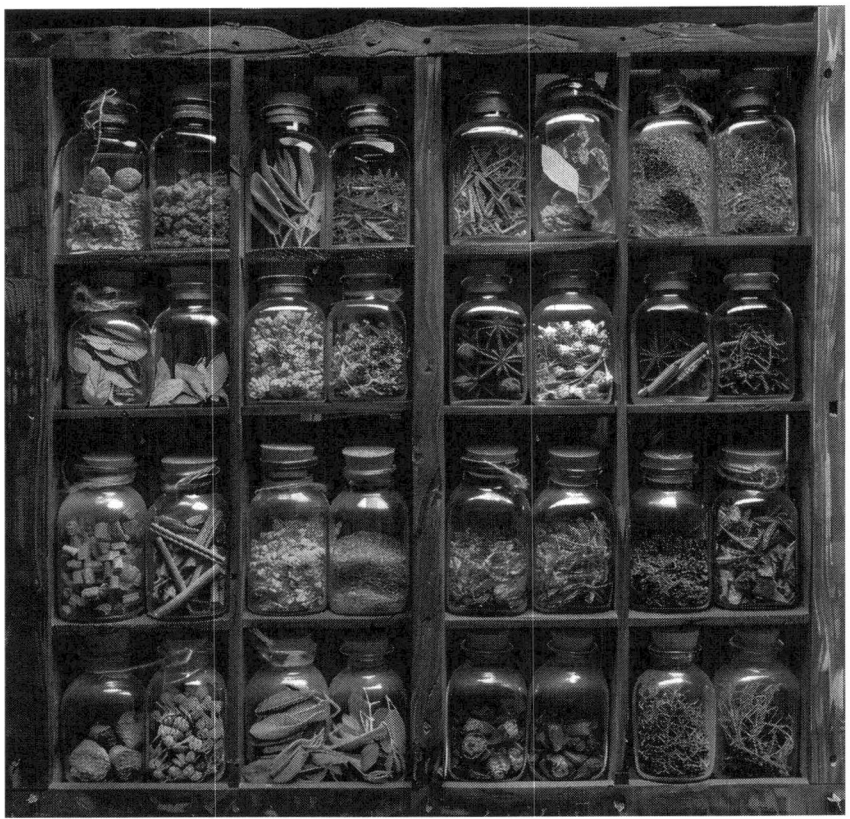

Fall, with its crisp air, vibrant colors, and the joy of harvest, reminds us of the cycle of life and the importance of nurturing and caring for nature. It is a time to reflect on the blessings bestowed upon us and to appreciate the hard work that goes into cultivating the earth. So, embrace the harvest season with open arms and relish the abundance it brings.

Here's a detailed step-by-step process for preserving and storing your herbal bounty:

1. Harvesting

- **Timing:** Harvest herbs early in the morning after the dew has dried but before the sun becomes too hot, as this is when their oils are most concentrated.
- **Technique:** Use sharp scissors or pruning shears to cut healthy stems, selecting those without disease or damage. You can harvest a large portion of your plant for annual herbs at once, but limit your harvest to one-third of the plant for perennials to ensure continued growth.

2. Cleaning

- Gently shake the herbs to remove any dirt or insects.
- Rinse them lightly under cool water to remove any remaining soil or dust, and be careful not to bruise the leaves.
- Pat the herbs dry with a clean towel or gently use a salad spinner to remove excess moisture.

3. Preparing for Preservation

- Remove any damaged or discolored leaves.
- For herbs with larger leaves, such as basil or mint, you might consider removing the leaves from the stems. For smaller, more delicate herbs like thyme, you can preserve them on their stems.

4. Choosing a Preservation Method

Drying

- **Air Drying:** Tie the stems into small bundles and hang them upside down in a warm, dry, well-ventilated area away from direct sunlight. This can take 1-2 weeks.
- **Oven Drying:** Place herb leaves on a baking sheet and dry in an oven set to the lowest possible temperature (usually below 180°F or 80°C) with the door slightly open for 2-4 hours.
- **Dehydrator:** Arrange herbs on dehydrator trays and dry them at a low setting (95-115°F or 35-46°C) for 1-4 hours, checking periodically until completely dry.

Freezing

- **Whole Leaves:** Place whole leaves on a baking sheet, freeze them until solid, and then transfer to an airtight container or freezer bag.
- **Ice Cube Trays:** Chop herbs and place them in ice cube trays. Cover with water, broth, or oil and freeze. Once frozen, transfer the cubes to a freezer bag.

5. Storing

- **Dried Herbs:** Store in airtight containers labeled with the herb name and date of drying. Keep in a cool, dark place. Properly dried herbs can last up to a year.
- **Frozen Herbs:** Keep in the freezer for up to 6 months for the best flavor. Use directly from the freezer in cooking.

6. Monitoring

- Check stored herbs periodically for signs of spoilage or decreased quality. Dried herbs should remain fragrant and retain their color. Discard anything that develops mold or an off smell.

7. Usage

- Remember that dried herbs have a more concentrated flavor than fresh. A general rule of thumb is to use one-third of the dried herb when substituting for fresh.
- Frozen herbs are best used in cooked dishes as they may become limp once thawed.

By following these steps, you can extend the life of your garden herbs and enjoy their flavors and health benefits throughout the year.

Case Study: Reflection on the Year's Therapeutic Journey Through the Fall Harvest

During the fall harvest at Christopher School, students not only create planters with autumn crops and blooms, but they also take part in transitioning their school garden from summer to fall. They learn about the specific needs of these plants and how to care for them during the changing season. This hands-on experience allows them to connect with nature and understand its cycles. Additionally, the activity serves as a moment of closure for the gardening season, allowing students to reflect on their progress and the skills they have developed throughout the year. It also serves as a new beginning, as they plant the seeds for a new season and look forward to the growth and possibilities it will bring. This therapeutic and reflective activity enhances their horticultural knowledge, fosters personal development, and provides a meaningful conclusion to their journey in horticultural therapy (Johnson, 2014).

CHAPTER 4
Aromatherapy in Bloom

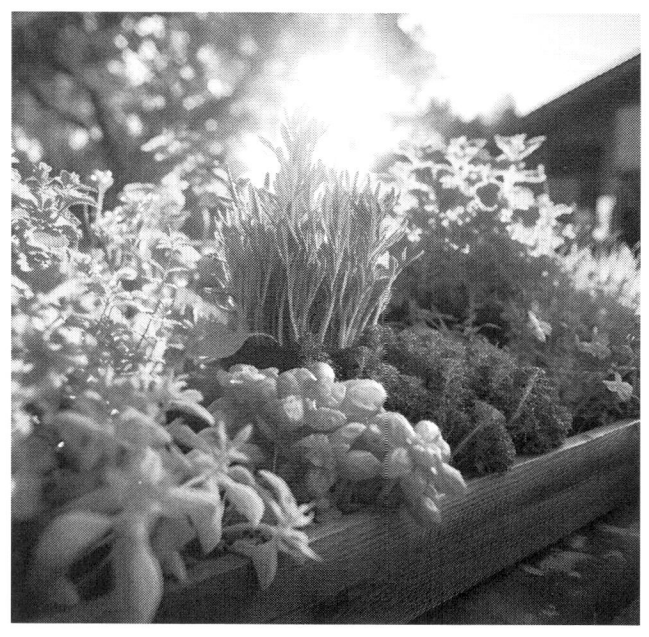

Aromatherapy can change brain waves and behavior. Research indicates that specific scents can reduce stress hormones, showing a strong link between the scents we breathe in and our mood and emotional well-being.

Just like medicine or meditation, scents have a calming and therapeutic effect. Transform your garden into a peaceful haven by growing aromatic herbs and basking in their calming aromas. But why confine yourself to the garden? You can bring aromatherapy to your bath, car, or workplace using herbal bouquets, infused oils, or homemade potpourri.

Herbal bouquets are a combination of elegance, beauty, and fragrance. They are visually appealing and release a delightful scent into the air. You can place them in vases or hang them in your home to create a calming atmosphere.

Infused oils are another way to incorporate aromatherapy into your daily life. You can create personalized blends by infusing herbs like lavender, chamomile, or rosemary into carrier oils such as olive or jojoba oil. You can use these oils for massage, add them to bathwater, or even apply them to pulse points for a subtle and soothing fragrance.

Essential oil diffusers have emerged as a revolutionary and innovative way to spread herbs' refreshing and soothing aroma throughout your living space. These diffusers employ advanced technology to disperse essential oils into the air, which helps to create an ambiance of calmness and relaxation. Essential oils are dispersed into the air as a fine mist using ultrasonic waves or heat to break them down. This mist permeates the air, providing a refreshing and therapeutic experience that reduces stress, improves mood, and promotes better sleep.

They are great for the colder seasons when the air becomes dry, acting as a humidifier in many ways; diffusers ease breathing by adding moisture to the air. They provide a natural remedy for congestion, allergies, and asthma.

With their versatility and ease of use, essential oil diffusers have become popular with many who want to enhance their home environment with natural fragrances and aromas.

Homemade potpourri is a simple yet effective way to bring the therapeutic benefits of scents into your surroundings. Gather dried herbs, flowers, and citrus peels, then mix them in a bowl or sachet. Potpourri can reduce stress, enhance sleep quality, and create tranquility by emitting its fragrance.

Whether in the garden, the bathroom, or your workspace, incorporating scents into your surroundings can profoundly affect your well-being.

SCENTED WONDERS IN YOUR GARDEN

Let's discuss a few favorite herbs that you can plant to transform your living, working, and private spaces into soothing havens of delightful scents.

Herbs for Aromatic Bliss

- **Lavender:** Lavender has a sweet, floral scent similar to lilac and is known for its calming and relaxing properties.
- **Basil:** Basil has a strong, spicy aroma similar to clove and is known to improve focus and concentration.
- **Balsam fir:** Balsam fir has a fresh, woodsy scent similar to

pine and is known to promote feelings of wellness and
vitality.

- **Oregano:** Oregano has a warm, spicy aroma similar to
  thyme and is known for its ability to soothe tension and
  promote a positive mood.

Creating Herbal Bouquets for Indoor Tranquility

Creating herbal bouquets is a great way to bring the beauty and
fragrance of herbs into your space. Herbal bouquets add a touch
of natural elegance to your home decor and infuse the air with
delightful aromas. Combining different herbs allows you to create
unique and personalized bouquets that suit your taste and preferences. Whether you have a garden full of fresh herbs or purchase
them from a local market, assembling these bouquets is simple
and enjoyable. Here are some tips for making beautiful and
aromatic hand-tied herbal bouquets:

- Select herbs such as fragrant rosemary, aromatic basil,
  and savory thyme to add delightful scents and visual
  charm. The different types of basil, like Genovese, purple,
  and spicy globe, not only add a pop of color but also
  introduce a delightful variation in texture.
- Consider the symbolism of herbs. Take rosemary, for
  instance, often associated with remembrance, or basil,
  commonly associated with love. Thyme, meanwhile, is
  frequently seen as a symbol of courage. As you assemble
  them, adding symbolism to your bouquets brings depth
  and significance to your arrangements, creating a
  beautiful story to share with loved ones.
- Create themed bouquets. For instance, a "Spaghetti

Dinner" bouquet with chives, parsley, oregano, and basil is perfect for a culinary-themed gift.

- Tie your bouquets with natural jute twine for a rustic look. This makes it easy to hang and dry the bouquets later.
- Consider packaging ideas. Pair your bouquets with related items, like pasta and fresh tomatoes, for a "Spaghetti Dinner" bouquet or homemade soup stock for a "Chicken Soup" bouquet.
- Remember, there's no need to follow strict rules of flower arrangement. Trust your instincts and combine herbs based on color, texture, and fragrance until the arrangement pleases the eye.

Case Study: How Aromatherapy Herbs Transformed a Space and Mindset

In Chelsea Clark's case study, she highlights aromatherapy's transformative power in altering her physical space and mindset. Essential elements in her routine include an essential oil diffuser and non-toxic candles, which she uses for relaxation and setting the mood. Her preference for dim lighting in the evening, aided by candles and lamps, further contributes to creating a serene environment conducive to winding down and drifting off to sleep. This approach illustrates the significant impact of aromatherapy herbs in enhancing the quality of living spaces and promoting mental tranquility (Dilger, 2023).

CRAFTING HERBAL INFUSIONS FOR THE SENSES

The ancient art of blending herbs for their aromatic and therapeutic qualities is a sensory journey that enhances mood and well-being. It goes beyond simply combining scents; it is a holistic approach that captivates all the senses and taps into the natural essence of herbs. As the herbs release their fragrances, the air becomes filled with a symphony of captivating scents, creating a tapestry of aromas that permeates the space. The gentle rustling of the herbs and the soft crackling of dried petals add a soothing rhythm to the process. The fragrant concoctions not only please the nose but also profoundly affect the mind and body, offering a sense of tranquility, revitalization, or invigoration. This ancient practice is a sensory symphony that uplifts the spirit and nourishes the soul.

Combining herbs based on their scents and properties requires understanding the principles of harmony and balance. Just like cooking, herbal blending involves knowing which scents go well together. Consider the strength and nature of each herb's fragrance, whether sharp, mellow, sweet, or earthy. It's also essential to understand the therapeutic properties of each herb. Some herbs may be calming, while others are energizing. The key is to balance these elements to achieve the desired effect of relaxation, energy, or sensory balance.

Creating unique herbal combinations can provide a wide range of sensory pleasure. Below are some creative herbal combinations for various purposes.

For relaxation:

- Blend: Lavender, Chamomile, Lemon Balm
- Effect: It calms the mind and soothes the nerves.

For energy:

- Blend: Peppermint, Rosemary, Basil
- Effect: It stimulates the senses and uplifts the mood.

For balance:

- Blend: Sage, Thyme, Lavender
- Effect: It harmonizes the mind and body.

These combinations provide a starting point for experimenting with herbal blends. You can adjust the proportions to your preference and enjoy the therapeutic process of crafting your unique blend. With that in mind, let's explore a few DIY projects using herbal sachets, potpourri, and infused oils.

Herbal Sachets:

- **Lavender and Chamomile Sachet:** Combine dried lavender and chamomile for a soothing scent. Place the mixture in small fabric pouches in drawers or closets for a calming effect.
- **Peppermint and Eucalyptus Sachet:** Mix dried peppermint and eucalyptus leaves for a refreshing aroma. These sachets can be used in wardrobes or cars.

Potpourri:

- **Citrus and Rosemary Potpourri:** Dry slices of citrus fruits like oranges or lemons and mix them with dried rosemary and a few drops of essential oils.
- **Floral and Herb Potpourri:** Combine dried rose petals, lavender, and tiny pinecones with a few drops of essential oil for a fragrant blend.

Infused Oils:

- **Calming Lavender Oil:** Infuse dried lavender in a carrier oil like almond or jojoba for a few weeks, strain, and use for massage or in a diffuser.
- **Rosemary and Thyme Cooking Oil:** Steep dried rosemary and thyme in olive oil for a flavorful infusion, perfect for culinary uses.

These projects allow for creativity and personalization, utilizing the natural properties of herbs to create various sensory experiences.

Anecdotes: Personal Experiences of Finding Peace Through Herbal Scents

Chelsea Clark's anecdote emphasizes aromatherapy's critical role in creating a peaceful environment. She incorporates aromatherapy into her daily routine by diffusing essential oils or lighting scented candles, which helps establish a calming atmosphere in her home. This simple yet effective method is part of her morning ritual, demonstrating how incorporating herbal scents can significantly contribute to a serene living space and overall well-being (Dilger, 2023).

THE THERAPEUTIC POWER OF HERBAL BATHS

Herbal baths offer a unique combination of hydrotherapy and aromatherapy, resulting in a soothing and holistic experience that effectively promotes relaxation, eases tension, and improves skin health. Incorporating herbal bath rituals for relaxation and stress relief into your daily life can significantly improve your overall well-being.

The use of herbs in baths has been practiced for centuries, and for good reason. When you soak in a warm herbal bath, the essential oils from the herbs are released into the water, creating a fragrant and therapeutic environment.

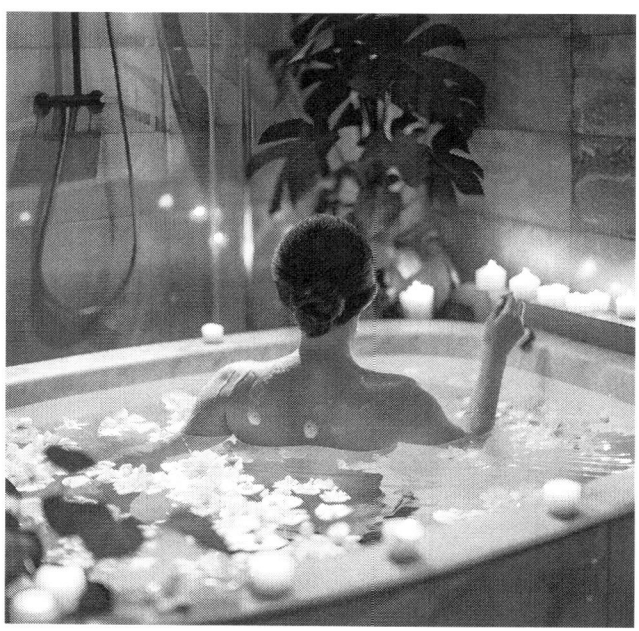

Hydrotherapy, or using water for healing, adds another relaxation layer to the experience. Indulging in a warm water bath can do wonders for your body and mind. Not only does it help to ease tense muscles, but it also stimulates blood circulation, leaving you feeling reinvigorated and at ease.

Aromatherapy, on the other hand, harnesses the power of scent to affect mood and emotions. The essential oils in the herbs have different properties that can help to uplift, relax, or balance your mind and body. Lavender, for example, is known for its calming properties, while citrus oils can boost energy and mood.

Below are some steps to create your perfect herbal bath.

1. To create your herbal bath, select herbs that align with your desired outcome. Some popular choices include lavender, chamomile, rosemary, and eucalyptus. You can also choose dried herbs or essential oils.
2. Combine warm water and herbs or oils in your bathtub. Allow them to infuse for a few minutes before getting in. As you soak, take deep breaths and let the soothing scents envelop you. Close your eyes and let go of any tension or stress. To enhance the experience, you can add other elements, such as candles, soft music, or herbal tea. These additional touches can help to create a serene atmosphere.
3. After your bath, take your time drying off and moisturizing your skin. The relaxation and rejuvenation you experienced in the bath can continue throughout the day, leaving you feeling refreshed and grounded.

Adding herbal baths to your daily routine can transform your self-care and relaxation routine into a sacred space filled with soothing scents, soft textures, and calming sounds. It allows you to disconnect from the outside world and focus on your well-being.

Case Study: A Journey From Tension to Serenity Through Herbal Baths

Sarah Voiles sought ways to better care for herself amidst her busy and chaotic life. She discovered the ancient practice of ritual baths and found solace in it, making it an integral part of her routine. Her first attempt at it involved a blend of pink Himalayan sea salt, lavender essential oil, and rose quartz, which created a serene and rejuvenating experience. This was not just a mere routine for her but a transformative process that brought her closer to peace and tranquility. Sarah's experience highlights the rejuvenating effects of herbal baths and how they can offer a peaceful escape from daily chaos (Voiles, n.d.).

CHAPTER 5
Healing Touch: Herbal Remedies for Body and Mind

Did you know that the Healthy Minds Poll, conducted by the American Psychiatric Association, projects a significant increase in stress levels among adults in the United States in the near future? The Healthy Minds Poll, conducted by the American Psychiatric Association, reveals that around 26% of participants expect to experience higher stress levels in 2023 than the previous year. This represents a noticeable rise from the 20% reported in the last year, showing a growing concern for mental health and overall well-being. As we delve into herbal therapies, it is crucial to understand this trend to explore natural solutions to counter the increasing burden of stress in our daily lives.

These findings have revealed that there has been a significant increase in stress levels among individuals, emphasizing the crucial need for effective and accessible solutions to support mental well-being. In recent years, herbal therapies have gained enormous popularity as a natural approach to managing stress and promoting overall wellness. These therapies utilize a variety of herbs, such as lavender, chamomile, and ashwagandha, which have been used traditionally for their calming and stress-relieving properties. By incorporating these natural therapies into daily routines, individuals can enjoy a natural and holistic way to combat the pressures of modern life and improve their mental health. By understanding the growing concern for mental health and exploring natural solutions, we can take proactive steps towards better-managing stress and improving overall well-being.

NATURE'S PHARMACY: HERBAL REMEDIES FOR COMMON AILMENTS

Nature's pharmacy refers to the vast array of herbs with remarkable healing properties. These natural remedies are effective in alleviating stress, anxiety, and insomnia. By harnessing the power of these herbs, individuals can find relief from these common ailments without relying on synthetic medications.

For centuries, nature has provided a vast array of medicinal plants, their healing properties cherished by cultures across the globe. Chamomile, lavender, and valerian root are well-known for their calming properties, making them ideal for alleviating stress and anxiety. Chamomile, specifically, boasts compounds that aid in relaxation and enhance sleep quality, making it a favored option for individuals battling insomnia. Likewise, scientists have found a link between the scent of lavender and reduced stress levels and increased relaxation. These herbs offer a gentle and natural solution, as you can brew them into a relaxing tea, consume them as a supplement, or incorporate them into aromatherapy practices without the risk of side effects from synthetic medications. By embracing nature's pharmacy, individuals can adopt a holistic approach to their health and find relief from these widespread ailments.

Crafting Herbal Tinctures and Salves

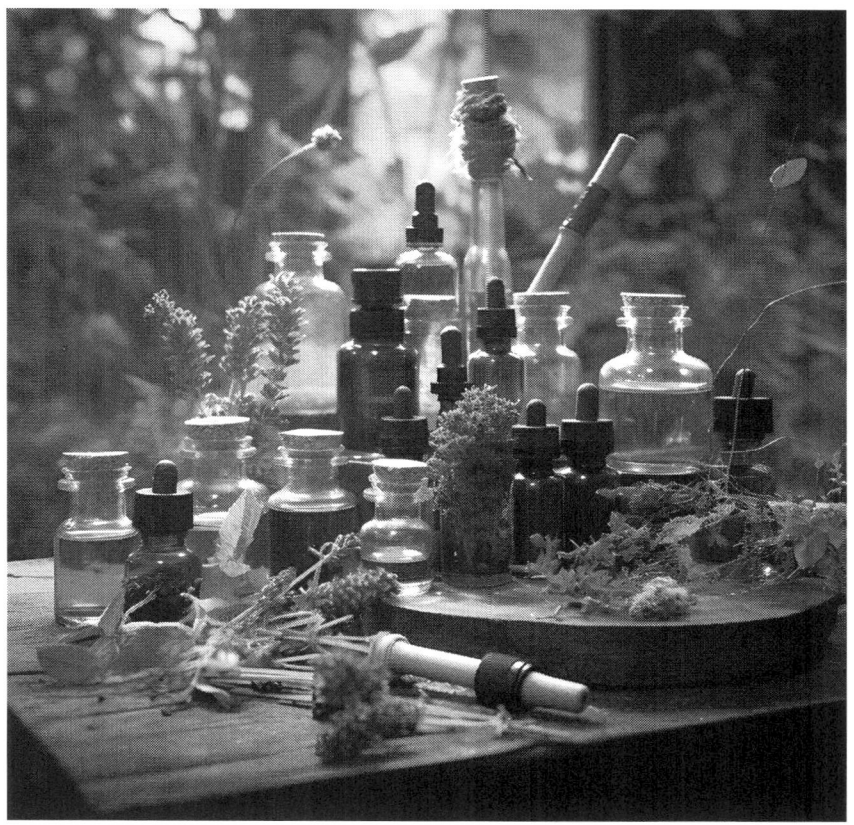

Crafting herbal salves and tinctures may appear intricate and even mystical, but it is straightforward and captivating. This age-old practice, rich in heritage, has been a fundamental part of traditional medicine for countless generations. It goes beyond mere herb blending; it is an artistry that harmonizes the medicinal qualities of plants with the expertise of extraction and conservation.

Salves and tinctures have a long history of use for their thera-peutic benefits. They offer natural solutions for various ailments —these herbal remedies work by extracting the active compounds from plants. When applied to the skin, salves provide localized relief and healing. In contrast, tinctures provide a more systemic approach to wellness when ingested orally.

Making salves involves infusing herbs in "carrier oils," like olive or coconut oil, allowing the beneficial compounds to be extracted and concentrated. This process often involves gently heating the herbs and oil together to encourage the transfer of medicinal properties. Once the infusion is complete, the mixture is strained and combined with beeswax to create a solid, easy-to-apply salve. The result is a topical remedy that can be used for various purposes, including easing skin irritation, reducing inflammation, and promoting wound healing.

On the other hand, tinctures involve using alcohol or a combina-tion of alcohol and water to extract medicinal compounds from herbs. Acting as a solvent, the alcohol draws out and preserves the plant's active constituents, ensuring their longevity for future applications. When taking tinctures, the most common method is to consume them orally. This can be achieved by putting a few drops under the tongue or diluting them in water or juice. This allows for absorbing the herb's therapeutic properties into the bloodstream, providing a more systemic and holistic approach to healing.

Crafting herbal salves and tinctures requires knowledge of different plants and their medicinal properties and understanding proper extraction methods and dosage guidelines. Careful atten-tion to detail and a profound sense of the transformative abilities of nature's healing power characterize the process. Whether you craft your herbal remedies or procure them from a reputable vendor, including salves and tinctures in your wellness routine can deliver a holistic and potent way to enhance your health and embrace natural remedies.

The following sections will explore two recipes for making your salves and tinctures. These recipes will guide you through the simple process of turning herbs into effective remedies. Whether you're new to herbal medicine or an experienced practitioner, these recipes allow you to embrace the ancient tradition of herbal healing and integrate its therapeutic benefits into your daily routine. It is essential to always consult a doctor before trying any herbal remedies.

Salve Recipes:

Calendula Salve:

- Infuse calendula petals in a carrier oil (like olive oil) for a few weeks.
- Strain the petals and mix the oil with melted beeswax until it solidifies.

Lavender Salve:

- Follow a similar process with lavender flowers.
- Once the lavender-infused oil is ready, mix it with beeswax, adding a few drops of lavender essential oil if desired.

Tincture Recipes:

Echinacea Tincture:

- Soak dried echinacea in a jar filled with vodka or another high-proof alcohol.
- Seal and store it in a cool, dark place for several weeks, shaking it daily.
- Strain and store the liquid in dropper bottles.

Peppermint Tincture:

- Use dried peppermint leaves and follow the same process as the echinacea tincture.

Not only do herbal tinctures and salves allow you to harness the healing properties of your homegrown herbs, but they also offer a creative and hands-on approach to self-care. By extracting the medicinal compounds from the herbs and preserving them in alcohol or oil, you can create potent remedies for various ailments. Whether you want to soothe muscle aches, alleviate skin irritations, boost your immune system, or support overall wellness, crafting your herbal tinctures and salves provides a personalized and sustainable solution.

Case Study: How Herbal Remedies Replaced Conventional Medications for a Healthier Lifestyle

This is an inspiring story from a clinic where the power of herbal nutrition and personalized healthcare was demonstrated. A severely depleted and unable-to-walk patient underwent a tailored program of herbs, supplements, and lifestyle changes.

Within three months, she regained her health and mobility. This case highlights the significance of proper health education and the potential of herbal medicine to impact personal health significantly. The patient expressed gratitude for regaining her life (Woman, 2024).

HERB-INFUSED NUTRITION FOR WELL-BEING

Adding herbs to your meals infuses them with natural compounds and nutrients that benefit your health. Herbs contain combinations of antioxidants, vitamins, and minerals, providing several health advantages, including reduced inflammation, strengthened immunity, improved digestion, and enhanced heart health.

Incorporating herbs into your meals offers a natural and healthier alternative to enhance your culinary experience. Choose natural oils or make your homemade marinades for meats and poultry instead of using dressings in salads to significantly improve the nutritional value of your dishes. Enhance your meals with a touch of elegance by utilizing herbs, whether sprinkling them on pizza or adding a hint of mint to desserts, pleasing your taste buds.

One of the easiest ways to improve the taste and nutritional content of your meals is by incorporating a variety of herbs into your daily diet. Herbs are an excellent addition to our diet, containing many vital nutrients and health-promoting compounds. Consuming herbs offers a range of benefits, such as immune-boosting vitamins and disease-fighting antioxidants, which help improve overall well-being. Whether you're a fan of the bold, fragrant scent of basil, the deep, earthy taste of rosemary, or the calming properties of chamomile, incorporating these natural ingredients into your meals and daily rituals can offer enhanced vitality, improved digestion, and a more balanced mood. Moreover, they can add depth and complexity to the flavors of your meals, making them more enjoyable and satisfying.

For example, adding fresh basil to your tomato sauce can give it a sweet and slightly peppery taste, while rosemary can give your roasted chicken a savory and earthy flavor. You can also use herbs to replace salt and other unhealthy seasonings, making your meals healthier and more natural.

Experimenting with different herbs and spices can help you discover new flavor combinations and improve your meal's nutritional value. So, don't be afraid to get creative in the kitchen and try new herbs and spices to take your meals to the next level!

Recipes for Herb-Infused Dishes

Fresh Herb Salad

Ingredients

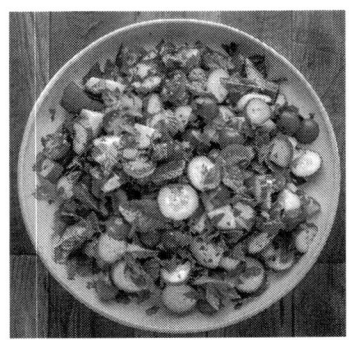

- 2 cups of mixed greens
- *These can be any combination of lettuce, chopped cabbage, or baby spinach you prefer.*
- 1/2 cup of chopped basil
- 1/2 cup of chopped mint
- 1/2 cup of chopped cilantro
- 1 cup of chopped cucumber
- 1 cup of chopped cherry tomatoes
- 2 tbsp olive oil
- 1 tsp lemon juice
- a pinch of salt and pepper

Recipe

1. Combine mixed greens with finely chopped basil, mint, and cilantro.
2. Add slices of crisp cucumber and juicy cherry tomatoes and drizzle with a light dressing of olive oil, tangy lemon juice, and even a hint of garlic for a burst of flavor. Garnish with edible flowers or add pumpkin seeds for an extra touch of seasonal elegance.

Vegan Pasta

Ingredients

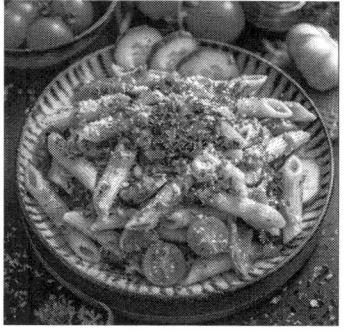

- 2-3 cups of cooked pasta
- *Choose the pasta you like best: penne, fusilli, or spaghetti. Follow package directions.*
- 1/2 cup chopped garlic
- 1/2 cup chopped parsley
- 1/2 cup chopped oregano
- 1/2 cup chopped thyme
- Pasta sauce
- *Choose a store-ready sauce or stew fresh, peeled tomatoes with oil.*

Recipe

1. Bring sauce to a boil.
2. Blend garlic, oregano, and thyme into the sauce and let it simmer for 10- 15 minutes.
3. Toss sauce with cooked pasta.

4. Plate and garnish with fresh parsley.
5. Add roasted cherry tomatoes, garlic, and a splash of olive oil to enhance the flavors.

Herb-Infused Mushroom Risotto

Ingredients:

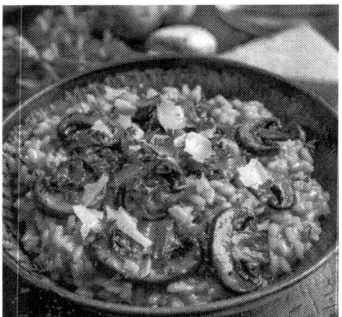

- 1.5 cups Arborio rice
- 4 cups vegetable broth, kept warm
- 2 cups mixed mushrooms (such as shiitake, cremini, and portobello), thinly sliced
- 1 large onion, finely chopped
- 2 cloves garlic, minced
- 1/2 cup dry white wine
- 1/2 cup freshly grated Parmesan cheese (optional for vegan option; can use nutritional yeast)
- 3 tablespoons olive oil
- 1/4 cup fresh parsley, finely chopped
- 2 tablespoons fresh thyme leaves
- Salt and black pepper to taste

Instructions:

1. Heat 2 tablespoons olive oil over medium heat in a large pan. Add the mushrooms and sauté until they're golden brown. Season with salt and pepper, then set aside.
2. In the same pan, add the remaining olive oil and sauté the onion and garlic until translucent.

3. Add the Arborio rice, stirring for about 2 minutes until the edges become slightly transparent.

4. Pour in the white wine and stir until it is fully absorbed.

5. Begin adding the warm vegetable broth, one ladle at a time, allowing the rice to absorb the liquid before adding more. Stir continuously.

6. Once the rice is cooked al dente (about 18-20 minutes), stir in the sautéed mushrooms, Parmesan cheese (or nutritional yeast), parsley, and thyme. Adjust seasoning with salt and pepper.

7. Serve immediately, garnished with additional parsley and thyme.

Herb and Cheese Stuffed Zucchini Boats

Ingredients:

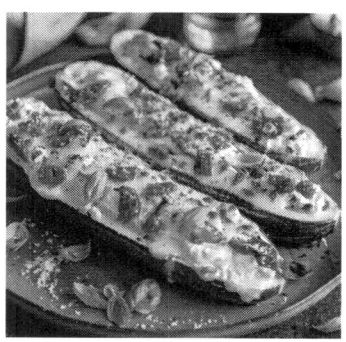

- 4 medium zucchinis, halved lengthwise
- 1 cup ricotta cheese
- 1/4 cup fresh basil, chopped
- 2 tablespoons fresh oregano, chopped
- 1/4 cup sun-dried tomatoes, chopped
- 2 cloves garlic, minced
- 1 cup shredded mozzarella cheese
- Salt and black pepper to taste
- Olive oil for drizzling

Instructions:

1. Preheat the oven to 375°F (190°C). Scoop out the center of each zucchini half to create a "boat."
2. In a bowl, mix ricotta, basil, oregano, sun-dried tomatoes, garlic, salt, and pepper.
3. Fill each zucchini boat with the herb-cheese mixture. Place the stuffed zucchini on a baking sheet.
4. Top with shredded mozzarella cheese and drizzle with olive oil.
5. Bake for 25-30 minutes until the cheese is bubbly and golden and the zucchini is tender.
6. Serve hot, garnished with additional basil and oregano.

Creamy Herb and Garlic Pasta

Ingredients:

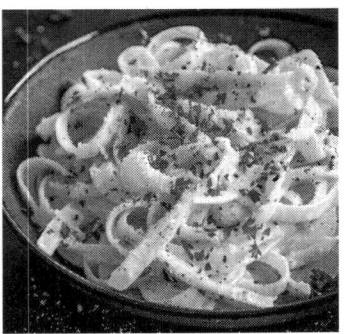

- 8 oz (225 g) pasta (such as fettuccine or spaghetti)
- 1 cup heavy cream (or coconut milk for a vegan option)
- 1/2 cup fresh parsley, chopped
- 1/4 cup fresh chives, chopped
- 3 cloves garlic, minced
- 2 tablespoons olive oil
- 1 lemon, zested and juiced
- Salt and black pepper to taste
- Red pepper flakes for garnish (optional)

Instructions:

1. Cook the pasta according to package instructions until al dente. Drain, reserving 1 cup of pasta water.
2. In a large skillet, heat the olive oil over medium heat. Add the garlic and sauté until fragrant, about 1 minute.
3. Lower the heat and add the heavy cream (or coconut milk), lemon zest, and lemon juice. Stir to combine.
4. Add the cooked pasta to the skillet, tossing to coat with the sauce. If the sauce is too thick, add some reserved pasta water until you reach the desired consistency.
5. Stir in the parsley and chives, and season with salt and black pepper.
6. Serve immediately, garnished with red pepper flakes if desired.

Pair these dishes with a cup of herbal tea that complements their flavors. For the salad, a mint or chamomile tea would be refreshing. A basil or rosemary tea can create a harmonious dining experience for the pasta.

Anecdotes: Transformative Effects of Herbal Nutrition on Personal Health

Cinnamon and sage are both well-known for their incredible health benefits. Cinnamon is widely recognized for its role in lowering blood sugar and fighting inflammation. This is due to its active compound, cinnamaldehyde, which has medicinal effects like lowering cholesterol and triglycerides and is a powerful antioxidant.

On the other hand, sage is well-known for its brain-boosting properties, which can significantly benefit individuals with Alzheimer's. Its distinct scent adds a refreshing touch to any space. The herb's ability to hinder the breakdown of acetylcholine, an essential neurotransmitter in the brain, achieves this. Both cinnamon and sage have a rich historical background in healing practices, and their health-promoting properties continue to be supported by modern research (Leech, 2017).

In addition to their advantages, both cinnamon and sage possess antioxidant properties. Antioxidants are essential for combating oxidative stress and ensuring the well-being of cells and tissues. With its high concentration of polyphenols, cinnamon is packed with potent antioxidants that neutralize harmful free radicals in the body. Conversely, sage is rich in beneficial compounds like rosmarinic acid and carnosic acid, both of which have been shown to possess strong antioxidant effects. These antioxidants offer protection against chronic diseases such as heart disease, cancer, and neurodegenerative disorders.

HERBAL FIRST AID: NATURE'S EMERGENCY KIT

Herbal first aid kits are essential for treating minor injuries and discomforts. They offer effective natural remedies, including essential herbs like arnica for bruises, calendula for skin problems, comfrey for wound healing, and echinacea for infections. These kits contain various forms of these herbs, such as tinctures, salves, and capsules.

In today's world, modern homes must have a first aid kit. This kit is essential for everyday emergencies, particularly in households with lively children or elderly family members. A first aid kit typically equips supplies for minor injuries and ailments such as cuts, burns, bruises, and headaches. These kits can reach a more holistic level by incorporating herbal remedies, enhancing their significance. Herbs, with their natural healing properties, provide an organic and effective alternative for many everyday first aid needs. By utilizing your herbal garden as a source of healing herbs, you not only make your first aid kit more sustainable but also enhance its therapeutic potential. Integrating natural herbs, tinctures, and balms into your kit allows you to harness the healing power of nature.

While modern first aid kits often rely on synthetic items, incorporating natural herbs and their derivatives, like tinctures and balms, can offer a more holistic and efficient approach to healing. Creating an herbal first aid kit provides a versatile, all-natural alternative to traditional first aid methods.

Herbal remedies have been used for centuries as a natural alternative to modern medicine. These alternatives are reputed to have comparable efficacy to prescription drugs but with significantly fewer adverse reactions. This is because herbal remedies work harmoniously with the body's natural healing processes rather than fighting against them, as some modern medicines do. Additionally, herbal remedies can help boost the immune system, promote overall health and well-being, and relieve various ailments.

From digestive issues to anxiety and stress, there is an herbal remedy available for almost any ailment. It is crucial to mention that herbal remedies require careful usage and guidance from a qualified healthcare professional. Improper use can have negative consequences, causing harmful effects and potentially interfering with the effectiveness of other medications.

Including herbs like aloe vera for burns, thyme for sore throats, lavender for stress relief, and calendula for skin irritations can address various everyday health needs. Next, we'll cover some natural quick remedies for common injuries that you can incorporate into your herbal first aid kit.

Quick Remedies for Common Injuries

Cuts and Scrapes:

- **Herb:** Calendula
- **Use:** Apply calendula salve or tincture to the wound for its antiseptic and healing properties.

Bruises and Sprains:

- **Herb:** Arnica
- **Use:** Arnica cream or gel can reduce swelling and bruising.

Burns:

- **Herb:** Aloe Vera
- **Use:** Apply fresh aloe vera gel to soothe and heal minor burns.

Headaches:

- **Herb:** Peppermint
- **Use:** Peppermint essential oil can be applied to temples or inhaled for headache relief.

Digestive Issues:

- **Herb:** Ginger
- **Use:** Chew on ginger root or sip ginger tea to alleviate nausea and improve digestion.

These remedies offer a natural and effective solution for many common injuries and ailments.

Case Study: An Emergency Situation Resolved Through Herbal First Aid

This case study explores the journey of a family medicine practitioner who embraced herbal remedies to enhance traditional healthcare practices. Initially, the doctor discreetly recommended natural alternatives for everyday ailments like headaches while following conventional medical protocols. The turning point came when the doctor openly integrated a holistic approach, combining herbal medicine with mainstream healthcare. People accepted this bold step, which reflected the respect the doctor had already earned. This story highlights the potential of herbal first aid and the importance of integrating alternative and conventional medicine for optimal patient outcomes ("The Emergency Doctor Who Teaches Herbal Medicine," 2019).

CHAPTER 6

The Meditative Garden: Cultivating Mindfulness

Have you ever considered the similarities between gardening and meditation? Both practices involve engaging in the moment and connecting with nature, establishing a sense of calm and a state of mindfulness. But what happens when we combine gardening with meditation? How does this combination enhance our mental clarity, emotional well-being, and spiritual growth?

GARDENING AS MEDITATION

Combining gardening with meditation enhances our mental clarity, emotional well-being, and spiritual growth. Gardening requires complete attention and focus, much like meditation. Engaging in gardening, we immerse ourselves in the present moment, appreciating the colors, textures, and scents of plants, which naturally quiets the mind. This process allows us to release stress and worries. By combining these practices, we not only cultivate our gardens but also our inner peace. Whether through meditation in the garden, using it as a cooldown after gardening, or gardening as a prelude to meditation, these practices synergistically enhance each other, providing a profound sense of connection with nature and self. Here are some basic examples of how gardening and meditation can be combined.

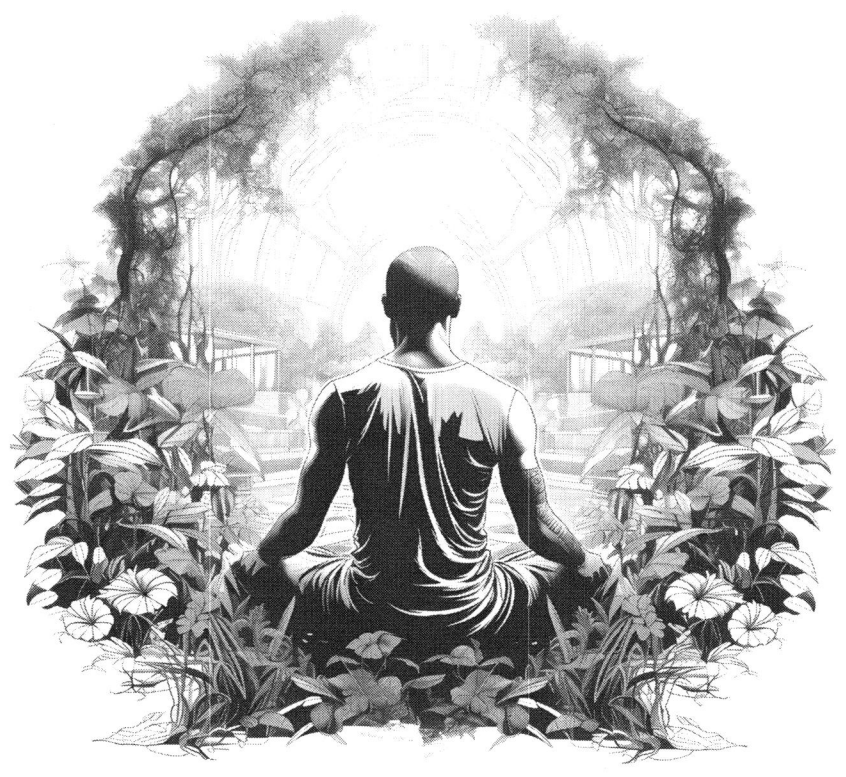

Mindful Practices in the Herbal Garden

1. Meditative Gardening:

- Engage in gardening as a form of meditation itself. Focus on each action, from planting seeds to watering, as a mindful practice. This approach allows you to connect deeply with the moment and the natural world.

2. Post-gardening Tranquility:

- After gardening, use the peaceful setting of your garden for meditation. Sit among the plants you've nurtured and allow the serene environment to enhance your meditation practice, bringing a sense of tranquility and grounding.

3. Gardening as a Prelude to Meditation:

- Start with gardening to clear your mind and prepare for a more profound meditative session. The rhythmic movements in gardening help release pent-up energy, allowing for a peaceful and meditative state to follow.

We foster a sense of interconnectedness with the world by tending to the soil and plants within our gardens. This connection is grounding and nourishing, cultivating a feeling of belonging and harmony. Gardening and meditation offer a unique opportunity for spiritual growth, allowing us to connect with something greater than ourselves. When we plant a seed, nurture it, and witness its development, it symbolizes all living beings' life force and interconnectedness. The garden becomes a sacred space, a sanctuary where we can commune with nature and access a more profound sense of spirituality. It becomes a place for reflection, introspection, and contemplation, enabling us to explore our inner landscape and connect with our higher selves.

Personal Narratives: How Mindfulness in the Garden Led to Profound Inner Peace

The Insight Garden Program in California's correctional facilities offers a compelling narrative of transformation and healing through horticulture. This program goes beyond traditional rehabilitation methods, using the act of gardening as a tool for inmates to learn and grow. Participants gain valuable skills and a sense of responsibility through tending to plants and engaging with nature. More importantly, they find a path to inner peace and mindfulness, which is crucial for their transformation. A poignant reflection from a former inmate encapsulates the transformative experience: "The garden taught me to cultivate more than just plants; it cultivated my transformation. It gave me the hope and skills to rebuild my life." This story illustrates the profound impact of connecting with nature in the most challenging environments, offering a beacon of hope and a new beginning (Chiocca, 2023).

HERBAL MEDITATION PRACTICES

Have you ever tried guided herbal meditations? It's like taking a transformative journey through the healing power of plants. By directing our attention towards various herbs, these meditations enable us to delve into each plant's distinct properties and energies. This practice enriches our comprehension and admiration of herbs and cultivates a more profound bond with the natural world. Engaging in guided meditation with herbs can unlock fresh realms of awareness and perception.

Guided Herbal Meditations

Developing a guided meditation script focused on herbal awareness can be a profoundly enriching experience. If you're looking to create your first one, here are some steps to guide you:

1. **Choose an Herb:** Start by selecting an herb, like lavender for relaxation or rosemary for clarity.
2. **Set the Scene:** Visualize a natural setting where this herb grows. For lavender, imagine a serene field of purple blooms.
3. **Engage the Senses:** Encourage the meditator to deeply inhale the herb's scent, imagining its unique aroma.
4. **Connect with the Herb's Energy: Guide them to feel the herb's calming or invigorating energy.**
5. **Incorporate Therapeutic Properties:** Weave in the herb's healing benefits, like lavender's soothing effect on the mind.
6. **Create a Flowing Narrative:** Ensure the script flows smoothly, allowing the meditator to immerse themself fully in the experience.

Herbal-guided meditations offer profound mental and emotional benefits. They provide a peaceful escape from the stresses of everyday life, allowing individuals to find tranquility and balance. Focusing on a specific herb can enhance mindfulness and presence, enhancing relaxation and reducing stress. By engaging with the unique energies of herbs, meditators can experience improved emotional well-being and a renewed sense of harmony with the natural world.

Incorporating Herbs Into Meditation Rituals

Like our guided meditation scripts, when using herbs in other meditation rituals, choosing the appropriate herbs is crucial for obtaining your desired results, be it relaxation, mental clarity, or energy. Take, for instance, the soothing blend of lavender and chamomile, a perfect combination that promotes tranquility and helps ease tension. Incorporating the refreshing scents of rosemary or peppermint into your space can enhance focus and concentration during your meditation practice. And if you require an energy boost, consider herbs 'such as ginseng or green tea, known for their revitalizing properties.

Each herb's unique energy and properties can enhance your meditation experience. The focus should be establishing a harmonious environment that aligns with your meditation goals. You can incorporate these herbs in different forms, such as fresh plants, dried arrangements, or essential oils. The perfect herbal atmosphere can transform meditation and strengthen your connection with yourself and the natural world.

Once you have chosen your herbs, there are various ways to use them. Pots or vases can be adorned with fresh plants, bringing a touch of nature indoors, while sachets or bowls filled with dried herbs release a soothing aroma. Using a spray bottle, try blending the essential oils with water. You can create a rejuvenating mist enveloping you in a relaxing and invigorating aroma. Strategize how you place the herbs in your meditation space to ensure the even dispersal of their scents. Position them near windows or fans to allow the aroma to circulate. Visual elements such as herb-filled jars or potted plants can enhance the ambiance and create a more serene and natural environment.

Case Study: The Impact of Herbal Meditation on Mental Clarity and Focus

Engaging in herbal meditation can improve mental clarity and focus, providing various mental health advantages. Research indicates that engaging in regular meditation routines can lead to reduced stress levels, including improvements in conditions such as IBS, PTSD, and fibromyalgia. It also promotes improved memory and attention span, which is particularly beneficial in combating age-related memory loss and dementia. Moreover, meditation strengthens willpower, aids in the avoidance of detrimental habits, and enhances sleep quality. It can also play a crucial role in pain management, lowering blood pressure, reducing anxiety and depression, and fostering greater compassion. By integrating meditation into daily routines, individuals can achieve a more balanced mental state and improved overall well-being (Cultivating Health, 2022).

CREATING SACRED SPACES IN YOUR GARDEN

Knowing the many benefits of merging gardening and meditation, why not create a space that fosters both? Designing your herbal garden to be meditation-friendly can significantly enhance the connection between gardening and meditation. If you're in the process of establishing a garden or wish to change an existing one to support meditative practices, it's a worthwhile endeavor.

Designing a Meditation-Friendly Herbal Garden

In the following sections, we'll provide simple and practical tips to help you transform your herbal garden into a serene, meditation-friendly environment. These guidelines will assist you in making your garden a sanctuary for botanical growth and personal reflection. Let's explore some important guidelines for setting up your ideal meditation space.

1. **Personalize the Space:** Include items that hold sentimental value or inspire relaxation and introspection, such as photos, art, or souvenirs.
2. **Implement Soft Lighting:** To create a peaceful ambiance, choose gentle, calming lighting options, like LED lights in soft colors or natural sunlight.
3. **Keep It Clean and Uncluttered:** A tidy and organized space promotes a clear and focused mind, essential for meditation.
4. **Comfortable Seating:** Ensure you have a comfortable place to sit or lie down, such as a cushion, chair, or yoga mat.
5. **Add Relaxing Sounds:** Consider incorporating soft music, nature sounds, or a noise machine to help you focus and relax.
6. **Accessible and Adaptable:** Make sure you have a meditation space that is accessible and adaptable to your changing needs or moods.

By keeping these tips in mind while planning your meditation herbal garden space, you can add an element of ease to the process while also enjoying the opportunity for fun and creativity. Embrace the joy of the planning phase and design stage, knowing that you will soon transform your garden meditation space into a haven of tranquility. Let's explore how your herbal garden can enrich your meditation practice.

- **A Quiet and Comfortable Area:** Design your garden to be free from distractions and noise, providing a sense of calm and tranquility.
- **Incorporated Elements of Nature:** Your herbs, plants, and other natural objects can enhance the calming atmosphere and connect you with the natural world.
- **Enjoy Soothing Aromas:** As mentioned in Chapter 4, integrating relaxing scents can create a serene environment. You can use the natural scents of your herbs or opt for candles, essential oils, or incense for a holistic approach. Store-bought options often offer unique combinations of herbs and aromas you may not have access to or know about.
- **Establishing a Focal Point:** Having a central point, such as a statue, candle, or piece of art, can aid in concentration during meditation. A plant or the entire bed could be a focal point in an herbal garden. Using plants adds a deeper connection with nature, as you'll focus on a living thing you've nurtured from a seedling.

Rituals for Connecting With Nature

Once you have set up your garden and are ready to embark on your herbal meditation journey, creating a meditation routine allows you to explore what works best for you and fully reap the benefits of your space. Focusing your garden meditation on specific rituals and routines can amplify your experiences and achieve stress relief, balance, a deeper connection with nature, or mindfulness. You can maintain a dynamic and gratifying practice by including personalized meditation rituals in your garden that align with your specific requirements, seasonal variations, or weekly plans.

Throughout history, experts have meticulously documented and passed down a variety of meditation techniques. These techniques have gained worldwide popularity as experts have proven their effectiveness in achieving their intended purposes. One example is the *Vipassana* technique, developed by S. N. Goenka, which emphasizes mindfulness and self-observation. In India, cultural practices like *Yoga Nidra* offer profound relaxation while maintaining awareness. In an herbal garden, it is easy to recreate the Japanese practice of *Shinrin-yoku*, which involves immersing oneself in nature. While these established techniques serve as a solid foundation, designing personalized techniques and rituals can be even more fulfilling.

By creating your meditation techniques and rituals, you can experience a more profound sense of fulfillment, allowing you to adapt your practice to align perfectly with your unique needs and preferences. To enhance your experience, you can integrate techniques that deeply resonate with you, such as tailored breathing exercises, affirmations, or visualizations. For example, you may focus on a particular intention or goal during your meditation, using mantras or visualizations to reinforce it. If you want to find the ideal meditation position for your practice, don't hesitate to experiment with different options, like sitting, lying down, or walking. Personalizing your meditation practice can deepen your connection with yourself and enhance the benefits you derive from the practice.

Consider selecting a time that aligns with your preferences, such as the tranquility of moonlit midnight or the enchantment of sunset, as each presents distinct meditation advantages. You can further enhance your experience by incorporating elements inspired by the ever-changing seasons, holiday motifs, or even the aromatic fragrances of various herbs associated with different times of the year.

Anecdotes: Stories of Spiritual Growth and Self-Discovery in Herbal Sanctuaries

In her botanical sanctuary, Katherine Yvinskas finds a profound connection with the *Dao*, the world's natural balance. Her living sculpture garden changes beautifully with the seasons, offering her a sense of paradise and spiritual fulfillment. This sanctuary represents not just a physical space but a journey of self-discovery and connection with the rhythms of nature. Katherine's experience, as shared, is a testament to the profound spiritual growth and discovery that can occur in such herbal sanctuaries, where the ebb and flow of nature resonate with one's inner self (Gladstar,2022).

CHAPTER 7

Herbal Alchemy: Crafting Elixirs for Emotional Resilience

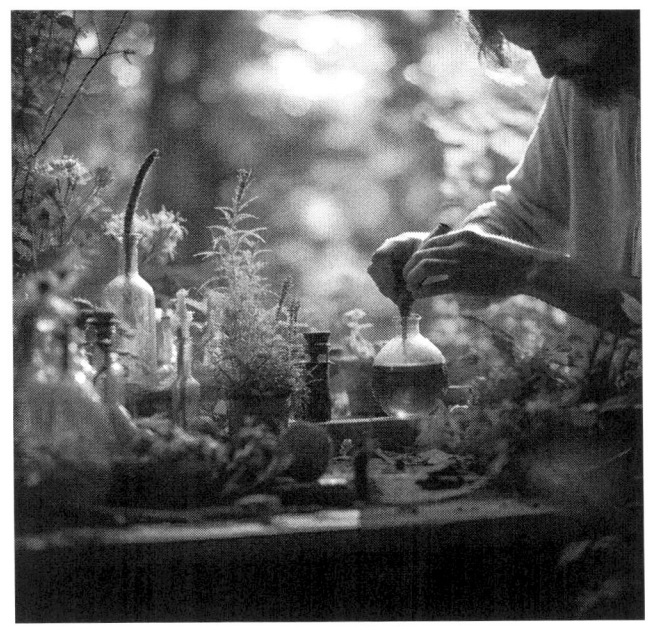

Herbal alchemy is an ancient practice deeply intertwined with the history of medicine and mysticism, offering a wealth of fascinating facts. During the Renaissance, people highly regarded herbal alchemy, viewing it as a science and an art that could transform natural substances into potent remedies. Alchemists believed in the philosophy of 'as above, so below,' which meant that they embraced the idea that the macrocosm, or the vast universe, reflected in human beings, the microcosm. Guided by this belief, they diligently worked with herbs, aiming to tap into cosmic energies and create potent medicinal concoctions.

These alchemists believed that by understanding the properties and energies of different herbs, they could harness the power of nature to heal and transform the human body and soul. They saw creating herbal remedies as spiritual alchemy, where the physical transformation of substances mirrored the inner transformation of the individual. They meticulously studied and recorded the properties of various plants, experimenting with different combinations and extraction methods to unlock their hidden potential. They filled their laboratories with vials, distillation equipment, and intricate diagrams depicting the connections between different herbs and their effects on the body. While their methods may seem mystical or even pseudoscientific by modern standards, herbal alchemists played a crucial role in advancing our understanding of medicinal plants and their therapeutic properties. Their work laid the foundation for modern herbal medicine and inspires researchers and practitioners today.

Emotional Healing Through Herbal Elixirs

Herbs for emotional balance and resilience can be a lifeline for individuals seeking natural remedies, especially those skeptical of traditional medicine or facing financial barriers to therapy. While these herbal solutions can aid in managing emotions, it's crucial to remember they are not replacements for professional medical advice or treatment. Using herbs from your garden adds a sustainable and health-enhancing aspect to your care regimen. You're taking steps toward emotional well-being and practicing eco-friendly self-care by cultivating and using these herbs. This approach allows for a deeper connection between nature and personal health, aligning with a holistic wellness lifestyle.

Several herbs are known for their ability to promote emotional balance and resilience. One popular option is St. John's Wort, which people have used for centuries to ease symptoms of depression and anxiety. Many people also use lavender for its soothing effects, as it can help relieve symptoms of anxiety and insomnia. Many of the herbs fall under a specific category known as "adaptogens."

Adaptogens are a group of herbs that aid in balancing, restoring, and safeguarding the body. These remarkable herbs can regulate the release of stress hormones like cortisol, which can become chronically elevated during prolonged stress. By reducing cortisol levels, adaptogens promote a sense of calm and balance in the body, improving resilience to stress and enhancing overall well-being. By possessing antioxidant properties, these herbs defend the body against stress and other environmental factors that cause oxidative damage.

Some well-known adaptogenic herbs include ashwagandha, rhodiola, holy basil, and ginseng. These herbs, which have a long history in Ayurveda and Traditional Chinese Medicine, are known to assist the body in coping with stress and maintaining optimal health. People can consume herbs in various forms, such as capsules, powders, or teas, and they offer many benefits.

These benefits range from promoting restful sleep and boosting energy to improving mental performance and bolstering the immune system. To optimize the effects of adaptogens, it is advisable to adhere to recommended dosages and rotate the use of different adaptogens every few months.

When addressing emotional resilience, it is vital to consider physical and emotional well-being. Emotional distress, which is often overlooked, can significantly contribute to various health issues. Herbs can play a critical role in supporting emotional resilience in diverse situations, such as fatigue, heartache, trauma, anger, loneliness, chronic illness, displacement, and nutrient deficiencies.

For centuries, adaptogens like St. John's Wort, ashwagandha, passionflower, chamomile, kava, motherwort, linden, and Albizia have been utilized to enhance mental and emotional health. These herbs help reduce anxiety, improve sleep, ease depression symptoms, and promote overall emotional health.

DIY Elixir Recipes for Emotional Well-Being

Emotional well-being plays a vital role in maintaining overall health, and using the natural power of adaptogenic herbs can bring about a significant transformation. Adaptogens such as ginseng, holy basil, ashwagandha, astragalus root, licorice root, Rhodiola, cordyceps, Schisandra berry, and turmeric are valued for their stress-fighting abilities and their ability to promote a sense of balance and tranquility. Below, you will find some do-it-yourself elixir recipes incorporating these potent herbs, providing a natural and holistic approach to supporting your emotional well-being.

Ginseng and Turmeric Tonic

- **Ingredients:** 1 tsp of ginseng extract, ½ tsp of turmeric powder, 1 cup of warm water, honey (to taste).
- **Instructions:** Mix ginseng extract and turmeric powder in warm water. Stir well. Add honey to sweeten. Enjoy this tonic in the morning for an energizing start.

Holy Basil (Tulsi) Tea

- **Ingredients:** 1-2 tsp of dried holy basil leaves, 1 cup of boiling water.
- **Instructions:** Steep holy basil leaves in boiling water for 5-7 minutes. Strain and sip slowly. It is ideal for evenings to unwind and relax.

Ashwagandha Nighttime Milk

- **Ingredients:** ½ tsp of ashwagandha powder, 1 cup of milk (or plant-based alternative), a pinch of cinnamon, honey, or maple syrup (to taste).
- **Instructions:** Warm the milk, then whisk in ashwagandha powder, cinnamon, and sweetener. Drink before bedtime to promote restful sleep.

Astragalus Root and Licorice Soothing Brew

- **Ingredients:** 1 tsp of astragalus root, ½ tsp of licorice root, 2 cups of water.
- **Instructions:** Simmer astragalus and licorice root in water for 15-20 minutes. Strain and drink warm. Excellent for immune support and stress relief.

Rhodiola Rosea Morning Elixir

- **Ingredients:** 1 tsp of Rhodiola rosea extract, 1 cup of cold water, lemon juice (to taste), and a spoonful of honey.
- **Instructions:** Mix rhodiola extract with cold water. Add lemon juice and honey. Drink in the morning for a mood-lifting and energizing effect.

Cordyceps Energizing Smoothie

- **Ingredients:** ½ tsp of cordyceps powder, 1 banana, 1 cup of almond milk, a handful of spinach, 1 tbsp of almond butter.
- **Instructions:** Blend all ingredients until smooth. Enjoy this energizing smoothie as a morning boost or pre-workout drink.

Prioritize consulting with a healthcare provider before beginning any new herbal regimen, particularly if you have existing health conditions or take medications. These recipes are intended to support emotional well-being and should be part of a balanced approach to health that includes diet, exercise, and stress management techniques.

Case Study: Transformative Effects of Herbal Elixirs on Emotional Health

A case study conducted by McIntyre et al. (2015) explored the effects of herbal elixirs on emotional health, specifically for people with anxiety. They conducted in-depth interviews and discovered three main themes: How herbal medicines are seen as different from pharmaceuticals, considerations of evidence and effectiveness, and the barriers to using herbal medicines. The study showed that herbal medicine is widely used, with reports suggesting that as many as 21% of individuals with anxiety disorders use it. These findings emphasize the importance of understanding patient beliefs and attitudes toward herbal remedies when managing anxiety.

HARNESSING THE POWER OF FLOWER ESSENCES

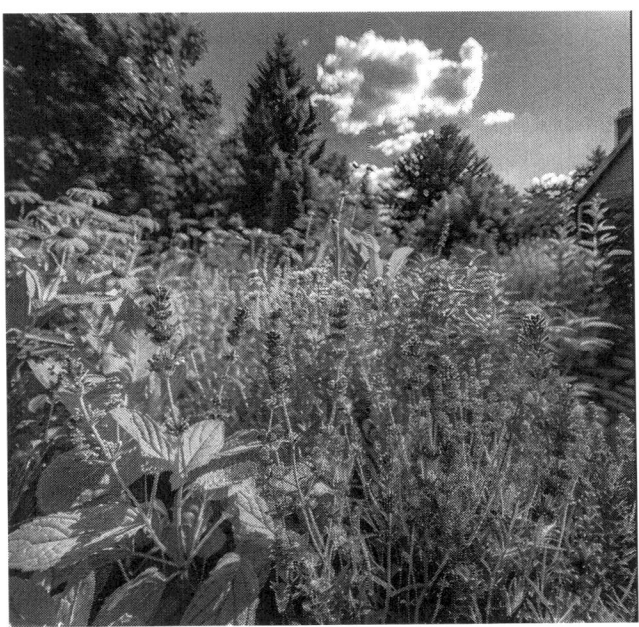

Flower essences are a unique herbal therapy focused on emotional and energetic healing. The significant distinction between flower essences and essential oils or herbal extracts lies in infusing flowers' energetic vibrations into water instead of extracting physical substances. This practice, steeped in the traditions of various cultures, gained modern recognition through the work of Dr. Edward Bach, an English physician, in the early 20th century.

The underlying idea of flower essences is that there is a strong link between our emotional and mental states and our physical well-being. Rather than directly targeting physical ailments, flower essences address the emotional responses and attitudes contributing to or resulting from health challenges. Flower essences are based on the idea that plants possess unique vibrational energy patterns, which can help restore balance and heal our emotional energy systems.

The process of making flower essences involves delicately placing the freshly picked flowers in a bowl of pure water, allowing them to soak up the energizing rays of sunlight or the soothing light of the moon. This process enables the flowers' energetic imprint to infuse into the water, creating a potent vibrational remedy. The resulting essence is preserved for long-term use by adding a small amount of alcohol.

Many believe each flower's essence has its unique energetic signature, addressing different emotional and energetic imbalances. For example, Bach flower essences, a popular type of flower essence therapy, have essences such as Rescue Remedy for stress and anxiety and Chicory for feelings of possessiveness and neediness.

When we take flower essences orally or apply them topically, we believe they work subtly, gently shifting and balancing the emotional and energetic patterns within our bodies. Flower essences should not be used as a substitute for medical treatments or interventions but rather as a complement, targeting emotional and energetic factors that can impact physical health.

Flower essence therapy is predominantly practiced by individuals who aim to enhance personal growth through self-care. This practice can provide individuals with valuable insights into their emotional patterns, help them release emotional blockages, and foster positive qualities such as love, peace, and joy. Regular use of flower essences has been shown to support overall well-being and contribute to a greater sense of emotional harmony and balance.

Although flower essences are generally safe, seeking guidance from a qualified practitioner before starting any new therapy is advisable, especially if you have specific health concerns or are currently on medication. They can help you choose the most appropriate flower essences for your needs and ensure their safe and effective use.

Creating Personalized Flower Essence Blends

Below is a step-by-step guide for beginners interested in herbal gardening and therapeutics.

Step 1: Selecting the Right Flowers

- Choose flowers that resonate with the emotional or spiritual healing you seek. Early morning is the best time to pick flowers when their energy is most potent.

- Use flowers from your garden or a natural environment free from pesticides and pollutants.
- It's essential to pick the flowers without directly touching them. Use a leaf or a piece of the stem to lift the flower, maintaining its pure, energetic essence.

Step 2: Preparing the Water

- Fill a clear glass bowl with natural water. The bowl should be wide enough to spread the flowers on the water's surface.
- Choose a sunny spot where the bowl can sit undisturbed for a few hours. This spot should be peaceful, free from foot traffic and strong winds.

Step 3: Infusing the Flowers

- Gently place the flowers on the water's surface, covering as much of it as possible without overcrowding.
- Allow the bowl to sit in direct sunlight for three to four hours. This process allows the energy of the flowers to be transferred into the water, creating a mother essence.

Step 4: Preserving the Essence

- After the infusion, use a twig or a leaf to remove the flowers from the water.
- Pour the water (now a mother essence) into a sterilized glass bottle. Add an equal amount of brandy or apple cider vinegar as a preservative. If you want a version without alcohol, you can substitute it with vegetable glycerin.

Step 5: Storing the Essence

- Label the bottle with the flower's name and the date of preparation.
- Store the bottle in a cool, dark place. The essence can be kept for several years if stored properly.

Step 6: Diluting the Essence for Use

- To use the essence, you'll need to dilute it further. Mix two drops of the mother essence into a 30 ml dropper bottle filled with half brandy or apple cider vinegar and half spring water.
- This diluted mixture is what you will use directly.

Step 7: Using the Flower Essence

- The general dosage is four drops four times a day. You can take it directly under the tongue or add it to a glass of water.
- You can apply it topically, add it to bathwater, or use it in a spray bottle to mist your aura.

Remember, creating and using flower essences is as much an art as a science. Trust your intuition and your connection with the plants. This process allows you to harness the subtle energies of nature for emotional and spiritual healing.

Anecdotes: Emotional Breakthroughs Facilitated by Flower Essence Therapy

In holistic healing, flower essence therapy, also known as flower essence alchemy, is increasingly recognized for its profound impact on emotional breakthroughs. This therapy works on all four levels of being: emotional, mental, physical, and spiritual. It involves the therapeutic use of flower essences to address deep-seated beliefs, unhealthy patterns, and emotional wounds, often rooted in childhood or past life. This therapy aims to facilitate the release of old, limiting beliefs and emotional patterns, empowering individuals to make healthier life choices and achieve emotional freedom. By integrating flower essence alchemy, individuals can journey towards embodying their highest selves and living fully in the present moment (Carrey, n.d.).

THE ART OF HERBAL TEA BLENDING FOR MOOD ENHANCEMENT

Crafting tea has a rich history and is deeply rooted in various cultures worldwide. At present, there are over countless blends of tea, each distinct in flavor and origin. Tea originated in ancient China, where it was initially consumed for its medicinal properties. The Chinese developed intricate techniques for growing and processing tea leaves and the art of brewing and serving tea. From China, the art of tea drinking made its way to various corners of Asia, such as Japan, India, and Korea. Each country, in turn, infused its distinct techniques and customs into the practice. In the West, tea gained popularity during the 17th century, particularly in Britain, where elaborate tea ceremonies and rituals were established.

Today, there are countless varieties of tea, ranging from black, green, white, oolong, and herbal teas. Each tea's flavor is individualistic, as it is shaped by elements such as the region of origin, altitude, soil quality, climate, and the techniques used during processing. Tea enthusiasts and connoisseurs appreciate different teas' intricacies, exploring flavors ranging from floral and grassy to earthy and smoky. The art of crafting tea continues to evolve, with tea masters and blenders experimenting with innovative blends, infusions, and flavors, ensuring that the world of tea remains diverse and ever-evolving.

Herbal teas are beneficial for your health and enjoyable to drink. These teas are made from various herbs, flowers, and spices, adding a delightful aroma and providing many health benefits. Take chamomile tea, for example, with its renowned ability to calm the senses and improve sleep quality. In addition to its refreshing flavor, peppermint tea is known for its ability to promote healthy digestion and provide relief from stomach discomfort. Ginger tea possesses anti-inflammatory properties and can aid in relieving nausea and improving digestion. With their distinct aromas and potential to boost well-being, herbal teas provide a flavorful and nourishing substitute for conventional caffeinated drinks.

Mood-enhancing herbal teas can vary in their flavor and aroma profiles. Some mood-enhancing herbal teas, such as chamomile or lavender tea, have a delicate and floral flavor, promoting relaxation and relieving stress. Others have a more robust and earthy flavor, like ginseng or ashwagandha tea, which can boost energy and improve focus. There are also teas with a citrusy and refreshing taste, such as lemon balm or lemongrass tea, known for their uplifting and mood-boosting properties. Additionally, herbal teas with a hint of spice, like ginger or turmeric tea, can provide warmth and comfort, enhancing overall well-being.

A vast selection of mood-enhancing herbal teas is available to suit individual preferences, each offering a delightful and distinctive flavor. Below, we have outlined a few simple steps to guide you in making the most of your freshly grown herbs and crafting your unique tea blends.

1. Choose Your Herbs:

Select herbs known for their mood-enhancing properties. Your herbs should represent you and your needs; choose the colors, scents, and tastes you identify with and, more importantly, the agents shown to combat your stressors. Headaches, muscle pains, and anxiety have known herbs to deter their effects; look to your resources and utilize the advice in this book. More importantly, don't be afraid to experiment, trust your instincts, and truly embrace your uniqueness in everything you create. This garden, these tinctures, this entire lifestyle is your own.

2. Gather Ingredients:

Prepare your chosen herbs, either fresh or dried. When using freshly picked herbs, thoroughly rinse them under cold water to eliminate dirt or debris. You can use a towel or a salad spinner to remove any excess moisture and ensure they are completely dry. If you're using dried herbs, there's no need to wash them.

3. Prep Your Herbs:

Next, remove the leaves from the stems if you're using leafy herbs like basil or parsley. Grasp the top of the stem with one hand, feeling the smooth texture, and then carefully run your fingers downward, sliding against the direction of the leaves. Discard the stems and keep the leaves. When using herbs like rosemary or thyme, you can easily keep them on the stems and remove them effortlessly when cooking or boiling.

4. Measuring and Blending:

Finding the perfect balance of dried herbs and water requires experimentation with different ratios to achieve the desired flavor and strength. We recommend using 1-2 teaspoons of dried herbs for each cup of water to attain the desired flavor. This differs as we all have personal preferences and will prefer different herbs.

Some herbs may have a more robust flavor, while others may be more delicate. It is best to start with the recommended ratio and adjust accordingly based on taste. Adding more herbs will intensify the flavor while reducing the amount will cause a milder infusion.

Remember to keep track of the ratios and adjustments made during the experimentation process to replicate successful combinations in the future.

5. Spice Enhancement (Optional):

Add elements like citrus peels or spices to enhance your herbs' flavor. For citrus peels, use a vegetable peeler to remove the colored part of the peel while avoiding the bitter white pith. You can add these peels to your herbs for a zesty twist.

For spices, you can experiment with flavors that complement your chosen herbs. Common spices that pair well with herbs include garlic powder, onion powder, black pepper, or red pepper flakes. Make sure to use only a small quantity of them so they don't overshadow the herbs' inherent flavors. If you want to add more drying time, transfer the items to a baking sheet and allow them to air dry in a cool, dry place until they are thoroughly dried, in case you don't need them immediately. For the best taste and to maintain their freshness, it is advised to keep them in airtight containers or jars, guarding them against sunlight exposure.

6. Grinding (Optional):

We highly recommend gently crushing herbs with a mortar and pestle to enhance the flavor and aroma.

7. Boil Water:

Heat water just before boiling. Different herbs may require slightly varying temperatures.

8. Steeping:

Place the herbs in a tea infuser or teapot. Let the herbs steep in hot water for 5-10 minutes, adjusting the duration based on your desired strength by pouring boiling water over them.

9. Strain and Serve:

Strain the tea into a cup. You can add some honey or your favorite sweetener as well.

10. Savor:

Take time to enjoy your tea. Focus on its aroma, taste, and calming effect on your mood.

Tea Rituals for Emotional Support

Tea rituals for emotional support involve creating a mindful and soothing practice around tea drinking. These rituals can serve as a form of self-care, offering a peaceful break from daily stressors. Here are some steps to establish a tea ritual for emotional well-being:

1. **Select a Calming Space:** Choose a quiet, comfortable spot to relax without interruptions.
2. **Choose Your Tea Mindfully:** Select an herbal tea blend that resonates with your current emotional state or desired mood enhancement.
3. **Prepare Your Tea with Intention:** As you boil water and steep your tea, focus on the process and let go of external worries.
4. **Create a Soothing Atmosphere:** To enhance the ambiance, consider dimming the lights, playing soft music, or lighting a candle.
5. **Engage:** Take a moment to engage all your senses as you sip your tea, noticing the aroma, savoring the taste, and feeling the warmth, allowing yourself to be fully present.
6. **Reflection:** Take a moment to reflect and relax. Utilize this time to meditate, ponder, or savor a moment of peace and serenity.
7. **Regular Practice:** Incorporate this ritual into your routine, whether it's a daily practice or a special weekly moment for self-care.

This ritual is not just about drinking tea; it's about creating a holistic experience that nurtures emotional health and resilience.

Case Study: Overcoming Emotional Challenges Through Daily Herbal Tea Practices

Keiko's experience with the traditional Japanese tea ceremony in Tokyo provides a profound case study of how herbal tea practices can help overcome emotional challenges. The ceremony is characterized by deliberate and mindful actions, providing her a much-needed respite from her high-pressure job. This daily tea preparation and consumption ritual became a therapeutic practice for Keiko, enabling her to find tranquility and presence in the moment. It illustrates how simple and consistent practices, such as herbal tea rituals, can significantly impact emotional well-being and stress management (Singh, 2023).

CHAPTER 8

The Herbal Home: Infusing Wellness Into Your Living Space

Continuing our journey, we will focus on incorporating aromatic herbs into our indoor living area. These indoor plants serve a dual purpose; not only do they enhance the aesthetics of our surroundings, but they also play a vital role in improving the quality of indoor air. Plants greatly enhance the air we breathe by absorbing carbon dioxide and releasing oxygen through photosynthesis. These plants help to increase air humidity by releasing water vapor from microscopic leaf pores, also known as "stomata." Although there are physical limitations to this natural exchange of gases, it still contributes to creating a healthier indoor environment.

INDOOR HERBAL GARDENS FOR HEALTH

For those looking to touch up our indoor living spaces with a bit of beauty and fragrance, indoor herbal gardening might be your next big project. An indoor garden can be just as fulfilling and thera- peutic as an outdoor one, more so for those of us who prefer the atmosphere and environment of our indoor living spaces to the weather and elements outside.

If you want to enhance the beauty and fragrance of your indoor living spaces, indoor herbal gardening could be your next exciting project. Taking care of an indoor garden can be just as rewarding and therapeutic as an outdoor one, especially for those who prefer our indoor spaces' cozy atmosphere and surroundings over the unpredictable weather and elements outside.

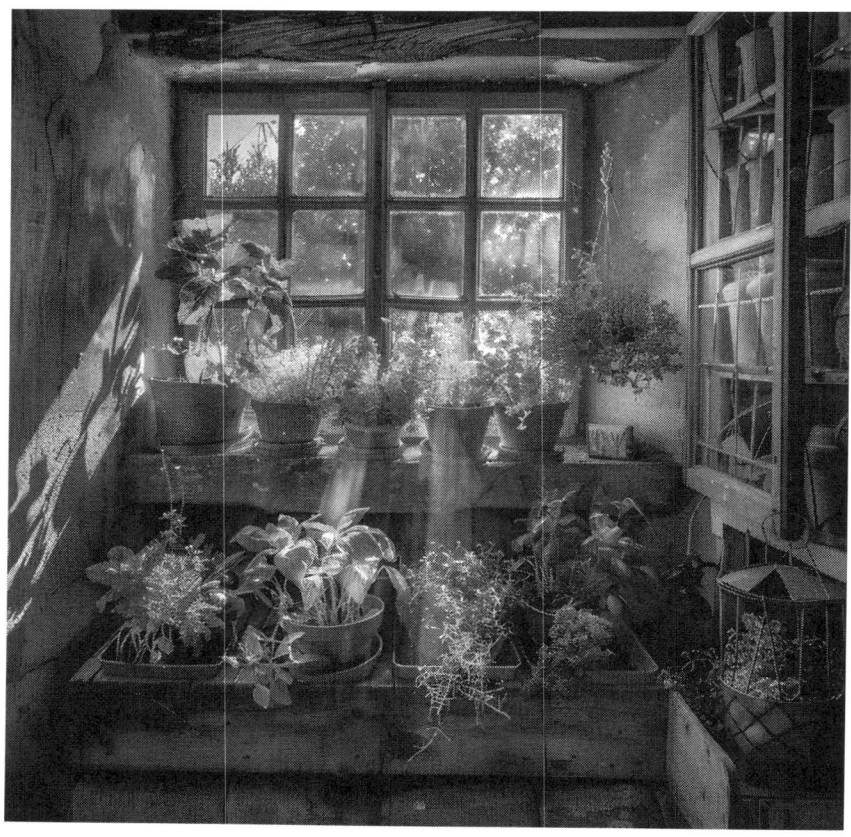

Indoor herbal gardening offers the opportunity to bring nature's beauty and delightful scents into your home, creating a genuinely distinctive and soothing atmosphere. With your indoor herbal garden, you can enjoy a year-round harvest of fresh herbs, regardless of season or outdoor climate. With portable lighting and grow tents equipped with air and filtration systems, you can easily recreate the ideal outdoor environment right inside your home. You can construct your dream indoor garden with enough space, this helpful guide, and a touch of creativity.

When planning your indoor garden, follow steps similar to those for establishing an outdoor garden, but with a few crucial adjustments. Here is a brief guide to help you get started.

Tips for Creating a Thriving Indoor Herbal Oasis

1. **Lighting:** Indoor plants rely on natural light from windows or artificial grow lights, so understanding the light requirements of each herb is crucial for their growth. Different herbs have varying light requirements. Some herbs prefer full sun and need at least 6-8 hours of direct sunlight daily. These herbs thrive near a south-facing window or under artificial grow lights that mimic the intensity and spectrum of the sun. On the other hand, herbs like mint and cilantro can tolerate partial shade and can be placed near an east or west-facing window. However, if natural light is limited, these herbs can still grow well under fluorescent or LED grow lights. It's essential to monitor the light levels and adjust accordingly to ensure that indoor herbs receive the right amount of light for healthy growth.

2. **Watering:** Indoor herbs typically need less water than outdoor plants. Over-watering is a common issue. Some herbs, like those native to the Mediterranean, prefer drier soil and should be watered sparingly. These herbs come from a Mediterranean climate and are adapted to survive with less water. On the other hand, herbs like basil and parsley prefer consistently moist soil and may require more frequent watering. Avoid letting the soil become waterlogged, as this can commonly result in root rot. A good rule of thumb is to water when the top inch of soil feels dry. It's also beneficial to use well-draining pots, preventing water from sitting in the bottom of the container. One way to provide moisture to herbs like mint and cilantro without over-watering is using a spray bottle to mist their leaves. Overall, understanding the specific watering needs of each herb is crucial for maintaining their health and preventing over-watering issues.

3. **Air Circulation:** Good air circulation is vital indoors to prevent diseases. A small fan can help, but avoid placing plants in drafty areas. Good indoor air circulation is necessary to prevent stagnant air buildup and promote a healthy living environment. Proper air circulation helps to reduce the concentration of airborne pollutants, allergens, and pathogens, thus lowering the risk of respiratory diseases and allergies. While a small fan can be an effective way to improve air circulation, it is essential to avoid placing plants in drafty areas created by the fan. Drafts can cause plants to become dehydrated and stressed, leading to poor growth and potential damage. Instead, experts recommend positioning plants in areas with gentle, indirect airflow to ensure optimal air circulation without subjecting them to direct drafts.

4. **Space Limitations:** Indoor gardens often have space constraints. Creative solutions like vertical gardens or hanging planters can maximize space. Vertical gardens are a great way to use vertical wall space. They involve growing plants vertically in specially designed containers or attaching plants to a vertical structure. This not only enhances the beauty of the indoor space but also allows for an increased number of plants to be grown. You can also consider hanging planters, which can be mounted from ceiling hooks or walls. These planters allow you to grow plants compactly and efficiently, using overhead space that might otherwise go unused. Various modular systems allow for easy customization and rearrangement of plants, ensuring that every inch of space is used effectively. These creative solutions enable indoor gardens to overcome space limitations and thrive in even the smallest areas.

5. **Temperature and Humidity Control:** Indoor environments allow more control over temperature and humidity, essential for healthy herb growth. In indoor environments, growers can manipulate temperature and humidity to establish the ideal conditions for healthy herb growth. Temperature control is crucial because different herbs have different temperature preferences. For example, basil thrives in temperatures between 70-85°F (21-29°C), while rosemary prefers slightly cooler temperatures around 65-70°F (18-21°C). By adjusting the thermostat or heating and cooling systems, growers can maintain the optimal temperature range for their herbs. Humidity control is equally important, as it affects the transpiration process in plants. Herbs generally prefer moderate to high humidity levels, typically 40-60%.

When the air is too dry, plants can experience water stress and may wilt or lose flavor. Conversely, too much humidity can create a breeding ground for fungal diseases. Indoor growers can utilize humidifiers and dehumidifiers to adjust the moisture levels in the air, ensuring a healthy balance for herb growth. With precise control over temperature and humidity, indoor environments provide a controlled and consistent setting for herbs to thrive and reach their full potential.

6. **Pest Management:** Indoor plants can still be prone to pests, but the types and management techniques differ from outdoor gardening. Pests can still be a concern for indoor plants, although the types of pests and the management techniques differ from outdoor gardening. Common indoor plant pests include mealybugs, spider mites, aphids, and fungus gnats. These pests can infest indoor plants by bringing them in from outside or through contaminated soil or plant materials. To manage pests in indoor plants, regularly inspect your herbs and plants for signs of infestation, such as yellowing leaves, sticky residue, or tiny insects. Isolating infested plants is an effective technique to prevent pests from spreading to other plants. Natural remedies like neem oil, insecticidal soaps, or homemade solutions made with water and mild dish soap can be used to control pests. It is crucial to strike a balance between pest management and the health of the plants, as some chemical pesticides may be harmful to indoor plants. Regularly cleaning and dusting the leaves of indoor plants and maintaining proper watering and airflow can also help prevent pest infestations.

7. **Soil and Fertilization:** Indoor herbs may require specific soil types and more regular fertilization to compensate for the lack of natural nutrients. When it comes to the soil for indoor herbs, it is vital to use a well-draining potting mix specifically formulated for container gardening. This will provide adequate aeration and moisture control for the herb's root system. Additionally, indoor herbs may lack access to natural soil nutrients, so regular fertilization becomes crucial. Using a balanced organic fertilizer can help replenish the necessary nutrients. Be sure to go with the recommended dosage and application frequency, as over-fertilization can harm the herbs' health. Regular monitoring of the plant's growth and appearance will help determine if adjustments to the fertilization routine are necessary. Also, consider alternate forms of development, like swapping soil for water-based hydroponics; you may find the options more suitable to your specific growing situations.

Best Herbs for Indoor Gardening

1. **Basil:** A versatile and popular herb, basil thrives in warm environments with plenty of sunlight.
2. **Mint:** Mint is easy to grow and used in culinary and medicinal preparations.
3. **Chives:** Chives can grow well indoors, adding a mild onion-like flavor to dishes.
4. **Parsley:** A staple in many kitchens, parsley can be quickly grown indoors. It prefers well-lit areas but can also tolerate partial shade.
5. **Cilantro:** Ideal for indoor gardening, cilantro grows quickly and adds fresh flavor to a range of dishes.

6. **Thyme:** A hardy herb, thyme is perfect for indoor gardens and requires minimal watering.
7. **Oregano:** Oregano is another excellent indoor gardening choice known for its intense flavor and medicinal properties.
8. **Rosemary:** Rosemary is a fragrant herb that needs lots of sunlight and can be a great addition to an indoor garden.
9. **Lavender:** Lavender can be grown indoors but needs plenty of light and good air circulation.

Each of these herbs has unique light, water, and soil requirements, but with the proper care, they can all be successfully grown indoors, providing a fresh supply of flavors and scents for your home.

Personal Narratives: Experiences of Transforming Living Spaces Through Indoor Herbal Gardens

This personal story showcases the creative and enthusiastic journey of an individual who transformed their living space into an indoor herb garden. Despite having limited space, they experimented with various plant projects, from growing peppers to attempting different broccoli varieties and even installing hanging baskets for lettuce. This narrative humorously illustrates the challenges and joys of indoor gardening, highlighting the importance of thinking creatively in small spaces. The experience epitomizes plant enthusiasts' dedication and passion for bringing nature indoors and creating a unique, green living environment (Curtis, 2023).

HERBAL HOME DECOR FOR TRANQUILITY

Adding herbs to home decor can provide natural beauty and therapeutic benefits. We've gone over one way to incorporate herbs into your decor. But it doesn't stop at your garden; you can use stylish planters or hanging baskets to grow herbs such as lavender, rosemary, mint, or chamomile. These herbs look visually appealing and release pleasant aromas that can help create a calming and relaxing atmosphere.

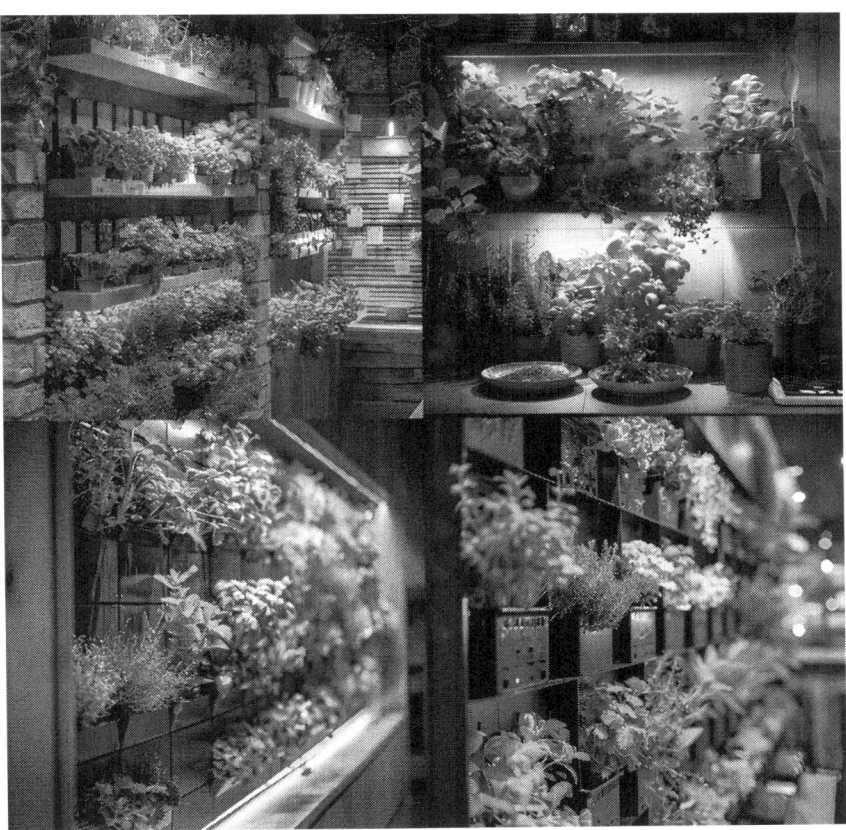

Many herbs have therapeutic properties that can benefit your well-being. For example, lavender is known for its soothing effects and can promote better sleep, while rosemary has been shown to improve memory and concentration. Use strategy when placing these herbs around the home and search for the arrangement, scents, and visual appeal that suits your taste.

The age-old trend of hanging dried herb bunches around your home is still in place and still provides the same therapeutic benefits as when your grands and great-grands did it. Popular herbs include lavender, rosemary, thyme, and mint. These herbs bring a rustic charm to a space and have several benefits.

Are you looking to relieve congestion and promote relaxation? Add some eucalyptus. A bit of sage is often used for its cleansing properties; many believe it removes negative energy from a room. When placed in well-lit areas or on windowsills, these herbs receive ample sunlight, allowing them to thrive and remain fresh. The vibrant green foliage of these herbs adds a lively and refreshing ambiance to any room, creating a soothing and natural atmosphere.

DIY Herbal Crafts for a Soothing Environment

Adding DIY herbal crafts to your home can create a peaceful atmosphere. One easy project is making herbal sachets. Fill them with calming herbs like lavender, chamomile, and rosemary. It's a therapeutic and delightful activity. Strategically placing these sachets around your home, whether in drawers, closets, or even under pillows, will infuse your living space with tranquility and encourage restful sleep.

An additional imaginative suggestion is to make your very own herbal bath salts. Mix Epsom salt with dried herbs like mint or eucalyptus, and incorporate a few drops of your preferred essential oils. These specially crafted bath salts not only emit a calming fragrance when added to your bath, but they also aid in reducing stress and relieving muscle tightness, turning your bath into a luxurious spa-like experience.

Want a quick way to refresh your room and fill it with the smell of your herbs? You should think about creating herbal room sprays. It's as simple as mixing distilled water with witch hazel and infusing it with essential oils such as lavender. This DIY spray revitalizes your living area, producing a soothing and refreshing ambiance.

You can enhance the tranquility of your home by engaging in various projects such as crafting herbal wreaths, making potpourri, or creating herb-infused candles. For example, a lavender wreath adds aesthetic beauty to your space and emits a gentle aroma that promotes relaxation. You can personalize the scent by building your potpourri with a blend of dried herbs, flowers, and essential oils to uplift or soothe your mood. Moreover, herb-infused candles can fill your room with a comforting glow and a pleasing aroma, providing the perfect ambiance for unwinding after a long day.

Not only do these DIY herbal crafts enhance the aesthetic appeal of your home, but they also create a calming and peaceful atmosphere. Engaging in the creative process allows you to create stunning, organic decor elements that align with your unique style and mood preferences while providing therapeutic benefits.

Case Study: A Home Transformed Into a Haven Through Herbal Decor

Adding herbal decor to your living space can make it more lively and vibrant. In a piece titled *How to Decorate With Herb Plants*, interior decorator Julie Nichols shares tips on decorating her home with herbal decor. She planted summer herbs in container gardens and brought the clippings inside to display around the house. She achieved natural fragrances throughout her home by placing the herbs in different rooms. Julie used everyday items like mason jars and tin cans to hold and display her herbs on counters and shelves. She also used vertical planters to decorate the walls. Julie's advice inspires those who want to transform their living spaces with the power of natural herbal decor (Nichols, 2017).

HERBAL FENG SHUI: BALANCING ENERGY IN YOUR HOME

Have you ever rearranged your furniture or adjusted the energy flow in your living space? If so, you have practiced the ancient art of Feng Shui. You may have heard of this term or its principles when someone suggested using a mirror to reflect light and make a small room feel bigger. This practice is known as the "mirrored illusion" or "mirrored effect" in Feng Shui.

Feng Shui, which translates to "wind-water" in English, is an ancient Chinese philosophical system that dates back over 3,000 years. It is based on the belief that everything in the universe is interconnected and that the flow of energy, or qi, can significantly impact our lives. Arranging our surroundings according to Feng Shui principles can achieve a balanced and harmonious environment that supports physical, mental, and spiritual well-being.

This practice of Feng Shui primarily involves analyzing the placement of objects, furniture, and architectural features, optimizing the room's energy, and creating a positive atmosphere. It considers factors such as a building's orientation, the arrangement of rooms, the use of colors, and the selection of materials. Decluttering and organizing our surroundings creates tranquility and energy flow.

While Feng Shui originated in China, its principles have spread worldwide, and many people today incorporate this ancient practice into their homes, offices, and other spaces to enhance their overall well-being. Applying the herbal principles discussed in this book to Feng Shui can enhance positive energy and create a healthier and more vibrant living space. Just as herbs have been used for centuries in traditional medicine to heal and restore the body, they can be applied in Feng Shui to purify and uplift the energy of a space.

Incorporating plants such as lavender, rosemary, or sage can bring calming and cleansing properties to a room. At the same time, herbs like peppermint or eucalyptus can invigorate and stimulate the energy flow. Combined with herbal aromatherapy, it creates a relaxing environment that promotes tranquility and balance. By integrating the principles of Feng Shui with the power of herbs, we can cultivate a beautiful space that supports our physical, mental, and emotional well-being.

Rituals for Harmonizing With Herbs

Various rituals can help harmonize energy with herbs. One common practice is creating an herbal smudge stick. To do this, gather dried herbs such as sage, lavender, or rosemary and bind them together with a string. While doing so, set your intention for the ritual, focusing on harmonizing and balancing the energy around you. Once the smudge stick is ready, light it and let the smoke fill the space, moving it clockwise to cleanse and purify the energy. As you do this, visualize the herbs' energy merging with the surrounding environment, creating a sense of harmony and balance.

Another ritual involves creating an herbal bath. You can incorporate Feng Shui into your bath ritual by arranging the herbs in a specific way that aligns with its principles. Start by selecting herbs corresponding to the desired energy or intention you want to manifest during your bath—for example, lavender for relaxation, rosemary for clarity, or eucalyptus for purification. Next, consider the placement of the herbs in your bath. According to Feng Shui, placing the herbs in a clockwise direction can promote positive energy flow, while placing them in a counterclockwise direction can help release negative energy. Additionally, you can position the herbs in specific areas of your bath to enhance particular aspects of your life. For example, placing herbs associated with abundance in the wealth corner of your bathroom can promote prosperity. Remember to take a moment to set your intention before entering the bath, allowing the herbs and Feng Shui principles to enhance your overall experience and bring balance to your energy.

Anecdotes: Stories of Improved Well-Being Through Herbal Feng Shui Practices

Combining Feng Shui practices with the healing properties of herbs is a great way to enhance your well-being and bring vibrance and energy into your living space or garden. In the article Spatial Alchemy: Changing Through Herbal Smoke, the author explores the ancient Chinese art of Feng Shui and how incense can be used to cleanse and harmonize the energies of a space. They explain that different types of incense can stimulate various energies and dispel environmental negativity. The author also mentions how incense is traditionally used in Asian cultures during funerals to facilitate the transition of spirits between realms. These stories and observations highlight the potential of combining Feng Shui with herbal practices (Herbalism, 2023).

CHAPTER 9

Gardening for the Seasons of Life: Herbal Therapy Across Generations

Have you ever considered how the timeless practice of herbal gardening weaves through the tapestry of generations, offering healing and connection across ages? From our ancestors' wisdom to our children's curiosity, how does this ancient art continue to nurture and bond families and communities in a cycle of growth and wellness?

Gardening has remained a beloved practice that brings families and communities together. From ancient civilizations to modern times, people have carefully handed down the ancient wisdom of cultivating and harnessing the power of medicinal herbs, benefiting the well-being of countless people. The act of tending to an herbal garden not only provides physical healing through the use of natural remedies but also fosters a sense of connection with nature and with one another. Children are often captivated by the magic of plants and their healing properties. They eagerly join their elders in the garden to learn and explore. This intergenerational exchange of knowledge and curiosity creates a bond between family members as they share stories, remedies, and experiences. Herbal gardens in communities serve as a common ground for individuals to gather, learn, and share their understanding of herbal medicine. This cycle of growth and wellness, deeply rooted in herbal gardening, continues to nurture families and communities by fostering a sense of belonging, preserving ancestral wisdom, and offering a holistic approach to well-being.

HERBAL THERAPY FOR CHILDREN AND ADOLESCENTS

If you're eager to get your children out of the house and in touch with nature while learning a valuable lifelong skill, there are plenty of child-friendly herbs and gardening activities. Everything from daily care and watering to labeling plants and charting growth. There are many fun, creative, and informative ways to get your children involved in your herbal gardening.

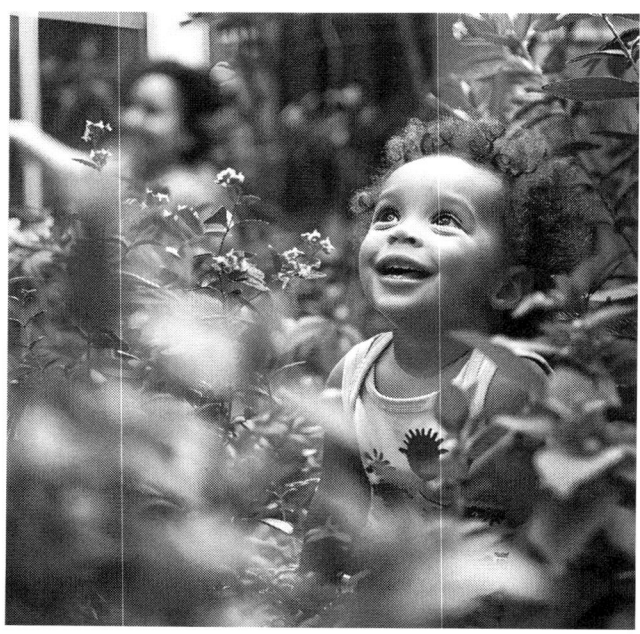

One child-friendly herb and gardening activity is creating a sensory garden. This involves planting various herbs with different textures, scents, and colors. Children can explore the garden using their senses, feeling the softness of the chamomile leaves, smell the fragrant lavender, and observe the vibrant basil and mint colors.

Another engaging activity is designing and decorating herb markers. They can use their creativity to make personalized markers for each herb, using materials like popsicle sticks, paint, and markers. This adds fun to the garden and helps children identify and remember different herbs. Involving children in harvesting and using herbs in cooking can be a great way to teach them about the practical uses of herbs and the importance of sustainable living. They can help harvest herbs like parsley and basil and then participate in cooking or making herbal teas using the fresh herbs they have grown. These hands-on experiences foster a connection with nature and instill a sense of responsibility and appreciation for the environment.

If your children are older and too preoccupied to get involved, you'll want to try a different approach. If you genuinely want to foster an interest in school-age children, try asking them to research climate conditions and what plants grow in what seasons or take them shopping for seeds and flowers. Give them their garden sections to experience the lifecycle all their own. For example, you could divide the garden into different sections and assign each child a plot to cultivate. Give them a variety of well-suited seeds and flowers for the current season, and walk them through planting, watering, and maintaining their plants.

Encourage them to research the different plants they could grow and challenge them to do it. This will enhance their understanding of the natural world and develop their research and critical thinking skills. Additionally, you can organize family growing competitions where each child showcases their section of the garden, and judges evaluate the growth and health of their plants. This friendly competition will foster a sense of excitement and engagement among the children as they strive to achieve the best results.

By involving them actively in gardening and encouraging their curiosity, you can nurture a genuine interest in school-age children and cultivate a lifelong passion for nature and environmental awareness. Another good book to add to your arsenal to keep your precious youths protected and healthy is "The Essential Guide to Natural Holistic Remedies for Babies." A must-have for newly blessed parents, uncles, aunts, and Godparents.

Case Study: Positive Impacts of Herbal Gardening on Children's Well-Being

Caroline, a holistic health practitioner, shared a heartwarming family camp story that emphasized the positive influence of herbal gardening on children's well-being. Her three-year-old child demonstrated an understanding of herbal remedies by suggesting using plantain to alleviate hay fever. This incident highlights Caroline's dedication to teaching her children and others about nature and self-healing through the use of plants. Her passion for empowering the next generation with knowledge about nature and self-care drives her work, showing the profound impact of herbal gardening on children's awareness and well-being (Woman, 2024).

Anecdotes: Heartwarming Stories of Familial Bonding Through Herbal Activities

A holistic health practitioner, Caroline shared a heartwarming story about how she and her husband successfully integrated their family and work despite the challenges of managing a busy practice, herbal business, and raising three young children. They involve their children in Caroline's work, such as foraging, herb identification, remedy-making, and healthy food choices. This imparts essential life skills to the children and strengthens familial bonds. One memorable moment includes Caroline's son assisting her during a school teaching session, an experience he thoroughly enjoyed. This narrative highlights the value of involving family in one's work, especially in herbal and holistic practices (Woman, 2024).

HERBAL WELLNESS IN ADULTHOOD

In modern adult lives, various common health concerns can be effectively tackled through the practice of herbal gardening and the use of herbal remedies. This can provide a sense of empowerment and self-sufficiency in managing one's well-being.

Through herbal gardening, individuals can easily access herbal remedies that address common health concerns. Having readily available herbs allows individuals to control their health and well-being, reducing the need for over-the-counter medications and promoting a more natural approach to healing. Gardening can be therapeutic, connecting to nature and promoting mental well-being. Overall, herbal gardening and remedies offer a holistic and empowering approach to managing one's health, promoting self-sufficiency, and fostering a sense of empowerment.

One specific goal you will achieve on our journey into herbal gardening is a sense of accomplishment. Successfully following the steps to assemble your garden and reap its therapeutic rewards will fill you with pride in your work.

Imagine the satisfaction of seeing your herbal garden flourish, with vibrant plants bursting with life and an array of aromatic herbs ready to be harvested. As you cultivate and care for your garden, you will develop a deep connection with nature and the earth, which can be incredibly grounding and rejuvenating. Tending to your plants and witnessing their growth will instill a sense of accomplishment and fulfillment, knowing that you have created something beautiful and beneficial for yourself and your loved ones. This sense of pride and achievement will boost your self-esteem and remind you of your ability to nurture and create amidst the challenges of daily life.

When the stresses of parenthood, school, work, or the isolation caused by lockdowns and quarantines become overwhelming, your herbal garden will provide you with a sanctuary of tranquility and respite. It will be a place where you can escape the demands of the outside world and find solace in the healing power of nature.

The calming fragrances, the opportunity to create homemade remedies and teas, and the satisfaction of cultivating your sustainable wellness source all contribute to the therapeutic rewards of your garden, providing comfort and peace. This nurturing relationship with your plants reconnects you with yourself and the natural world.

Let's explore and review a few ways we've discovered to integrate herbal practices into a busy adult lifestyle.

Integrating Herbal Practices Into a Busy Adult Lifestyle

If you're a busy adult looking to embrace herbal practices, one practical approach is making herbal teas a daily trend. Instead of reaching for a cup of coffee or a sugary energy drink, opt for a soothing herbal tea with various health benefits. You can prepare a batch of herbal tea in the morning and take it to work, sipping it throughout the day.

Another way to integrate herbal practices is by incorporating herbs into your cooking. Fresh or dried herbs added to your meals enhance the flavor and give them nutritional value. Continuously experiment with different herbs and spices to create new, delicious, healthy dishes.

Additionally, herbal supplements can be a convenient way to incorporate herbal practices into a busy lifestyle. You can choose or craft the supplements tailored to your needs daily to support your overall well-being. Just keep in mind to always speak with a healthcare professional when you plan on starting any herbal supplement regimen.

If you're looking for a social activity, consider joining a community garden to engage with your neighbors while learning to grow and harvest herbs. Community gardens are not only a fantastic way to socialize and connect with your neighbors, but they can also be a great place to learn and develop new gardening and social skills. Joining a community garden offers the opportunity to gain practical herb cultivation and harvesting skills. With more than just your hands planting, you'll have access to a broader range of herbs. It's a great place to trade and buy seeds and fresh vegetables, supporting the garden and your health at the same time. You'll participate in lively conversations with fellow herbal enthusiasts, sharing knowledge and exchanging tips, creating a solid camaraderie and friendship.

Community gardens are undoubtedly the best place if you prefer meeting new people. However, it's important to note that a community garden must not be a physical space. You can find countless herb enthusiasts like yourself on the internet and social media sites. Joining an online herbal gardening group can provide a wealth of knowledge and resources. You can connect with experienced gardeners who can offer advice and tips for growing herbs. You can share your stories and learn from others' successes and challenges. You'll also be helping the global community by teaching what you know to those who may be inexperienced.

Starting your online herbal gardening group can be a perfect way to bring together like-minded individuals who share a passion for herbs. You can create a space for members to exchange ideas, share photos of their gardens, and troubleshoot common problems. Social media platforms are also great avenues for connecting with fellow gardeners. You can join herbal gardening communities, share your progress, and engage in discussions with people worldwide.

While an online community may be the best for your busy schedule, we hope you'll consider exploring local community gardens, where you can meet fellow gardeners face-to-face if you can find the time. These spaces often host workshops and events that allow you to see the experts in action and connect with others who share your interest in herbal gardening. By embracing these opportunities for camaraderie, you can enhance your gardening practices and create lasting connections with fellow herb enthusiasts.

Finally, taking breaks and creating moments of relaxation can be an excellent opportunity to incorporate herbal practices. Whether taking a few minutes to practice mindfulness and drink a calming herbal infusion or using herbal essential oils for aromatherapy, these small moments reduce your daily stressors and silence them.

Caring for plants and maintaining a community garden is satisfying and physically engaging. It helps you stay active and enhances your overall well-being. In addition, community gardens enhance the local community by adding beauty to the surroundings and offering nutritious, pesticide-free food to those who require it.

A community garden is one of many ways to get social with your herbal gardening; another option is to start your social gardening group. You can shape the gardening social group in any way you desire, and it can be organized according to your preferred schedule. Extend an invitation to friends to lend a hand in your garden or offer your assistance in helping a friend start their own. There is no need to worry if your friend has never gardened before. Reading this far, you have absorbed all the necessary information to help them get started.

Case Study: A Personal Journey of Maintaining Health and Vitality Through Herbal Practices

In this case study, we delve into the personal journey of someone who has found a way to maintain their health and vitality through a simple yet effective practice of regrowing plants from kitchen scraps. The story revolves around an individual who, despite living in an urban area, has discovered the joy and practicality of giving new life to the ends of grocery store vegetables. They have cultivated a mini garden of garlic, ginger, celery, and more by placing these scraps in water and later transferring them to pots. This practice not only brings a sense of fulfillment and connection to nature, but it also contributes to a sustainable lifestyle. The story highlights the power of small, mindful actions in enhancing daily well-being and bringing a touch of greenery into urban environments (Curtis, 2023).

HERBAL WISDOM FOR THE GOLDEN YEARS

Focusing on herbs that enhance wellness and longevity is particularly beneficial for senior gardeners. As we age, our health needs evolve, making it essential to choose herbs that offer specific benefits for senior well-being. Let's explore a variety of herbs that are easy to grow and provide significant health advantages for older adults.

1. **Rosemary:** Celebrated for its potential to boost memory and cognitive function, rosemary is a must-have in a senior's herbal garden.
2. **Turmeric:** Turmeric, a powerful anti-inflammatory, is ideal for managing age-related conditions like arthritis.
3. **Lavender and Chamomile:** These herbs are excellent for promoting relaxation and aiding sleep, both crucial for maintaining good health in later years.
4. **Ginger:** A great digestive aid, ginger can help alleviate common issues like indigestion and nausea.
5. **Ginkgo Biloba:** Often associated with enhanced brain health, ginkgo biloba may be particularly beneficial for seniors experiencing cognitive changes.
6. **Sage:** Sage contains compounds that improve cognitive performance and may help manage age-related memory decline.

7. **Holy Basil (Tulsi):** With its adaptogenic properties, holy basil is fantastic for helping the body manage stress and enhancing overall well-being.
8. **Peppermint and Chamomile:** These herbs can soothe digestive discomfort, a common concern among seniors.
9. **Nettle and Dandelion:** Known for their detoxifying effects, these herbs support kidney and liver health.

These herbs can make soothing teas or infuse them with essential oils. Others can be used in cooking or made into herbal remedies. By growing these herbs in their gardens, senior citizens can enjoy nurturing and tending to their plants and access natural remedies that promote vitality and wellness in their golden years.

Adaptations for Herbal Gardening in Later Years

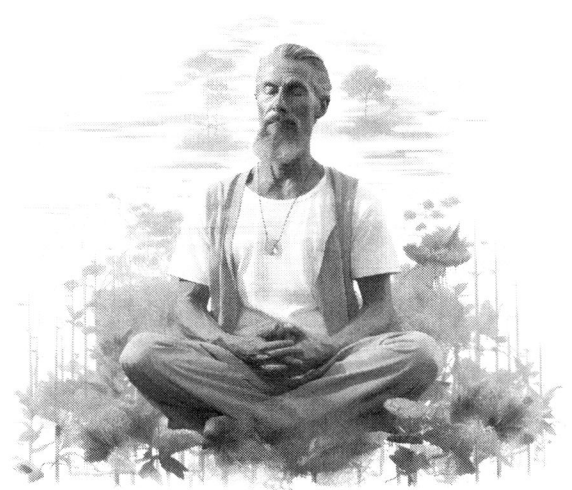

As we age, we must find ways to continue enjoying our hobbies and passions, such as gardening, while also considering any physical limitations or challenges we may face. If traditional gardening methods feel confining, there are several adaptations you can make to your herbal garden to accommodate the challenges faced in later years.

One option is to raise the garden beds to a comfortable height for you to reach without bending or kneeling. Raised garden beds or elevated planters can achieve this. Additionally, incorporating pathways or stepping stones throughout the garden can provide stability and support while navigating the space. Adding handrails or sturdy supports near plants that require pruning or harvesting can also enhance the ease of performing these tasks.

Last, ergonomically designed lightweight tools and equipment can improve your gardening experience by reducing the strain on your body. Look for tools with padded handles and adjustable heights to ensure a comfortable grip and proper body alignment. Lightweight tools are easier to maneuver and require less effort, making it easier to move around and perform gardening tasks without putting excessive strain on your joints and muscles.

In addition, it is advisable to use tools with extended handles or long-reach options to minimize the need for bending and stretching. Individuals who have limited mobility can significantly benefit from this. These adaptations will allow you to continue enjoying the therapeutic benefits of gardening and help maintain your independence and mobility for years to come.

Anecdotes: Stories of Enhanced Quality of Life in the Golden Years Through Herbal Therapies

The "Forget-Me-Not" garden in the UK is a heartwarming example of how herbal gardens can significantly improve the lives of individuals with dementia. Specially designed to engage multiple senses, the garden features scented flowers, tactile surfaces, and soothing sounds. These elements are thoughtfully integrated to evoke memories and stimulate cognitive function in dementia patients. The garden provides a tranquil and familiar environment where visitors can relive cherished moments from their past. Caregivers have observed remarkable moments of recognition and recollection in their loved ones, highlighting the garden's effectiveness in reconnecting individuals with dementia to their lost memories and providing them with joy and clarity (Chiocca, 2023).

CHAPTER 10

Beyond the Garden: Community, Sustainability, and Herbal Advocacy

Community gardens are much more than just areas for growing herbs and vegetables. They are vibrant centers of community interaction and environmental stewardship. Studies underscore the value of accessible initiatives like community gardens in promoting healthier eating habits. One such study found that after Hispanic farmworker families received education and support in organic gardening, they experienced a dramatic increase in vegetable intake: Nearly four-fold among adults and three-fold among children (Wu, 2020). These shared spaces are about cultivating plants, fostering community ties, and promoting sustainable living. For example, research shows that community gardens enhance neighborhood aesthetics and transform unused urban spaces into green oases, improving residents' quality of life.

Community gardens also function as educational hubs, providing opportunities for people of all ages to come together and learn about gardening, nutrition, and the significance of local ecosystems. Additionally, community gardens significantly contribute to regional biodiversity by providing habitats for pollinators and native species. The impact of these gardens goes beyond the plot boundaries, creating a sense of belonging, reducing crime rates, and promoting community members' physical and mental well-being.

HERBAL GARDENS AS COMMUNITY SANCTUARIES

Communal gardens are ideal community meeting centers ripe with opportunities for personal development, education, and building a more friendly community. This section will review some of these benefits, hopefully inspiring you to take community initiatives.

These social havens offer a unique platform for experiential learning. They provide a hands-on opportunity for individuals of all ages to gain practical knowledge about gardening techniques, plant care, and sustainable agriculture. Those participating in the program will receive education on the various plant varieties, including their growth cycles and the optimal cultivation conditions.

Community gardens often organize workshops and educational programs to teach participants about nutrition and the importance of a healthy diet. This enhances their understanding of the connection between fresh produce and overall well-being and encourages them to make healthier choices in their daily lives.

These gardens promote awareness of local ecosystems and their role in preserving biodiversity. Through interactive activities and discussions, participants gain a deeper appreciation for the natural environment and become more motivated to protect and conserve it.

Community gardens have many benefits beyond enhancing neighborhood aesthetics. These green oases not only transform unused urban spaces but also provide a range of social, environmental, and health benefits. Research has shown that community gardens promote social interactions and strengthen community bonds as neighbors come together to cultivate the land and share gardening knowledge.

These gardens play a crucial role in ensuring food security for residents, particularly in areas where affordable and nutritious food options are scarce. They provide a steady supply of fresh and healthy produce, thereby addressing the issue of limited access to such food resources.

Community gardens have been linked to improved mental well-being and reduced stress among residents, as spending time in nature and gardening positively impacts mental health.

Initiatives for Creating Herbal Community Spaces

Creating herbal community spaces can be achieved through a range of initiatives. One crucial step is to rally your green-thumbed troops. Look for locals who share your interests online and start community groups. Talk with your neighbors about your plans, invite them to join you, and ask for their suggestions. Building your community of garden lovers establishes a foundation for your community garden before it even exists. This lightens the physical load on you and the resources required of you alone, but more importantly, it gets the word out. A good starting initiative is to establish community gardens dedicated to growing medicinal herbs. These gardens can serve as educational and therapeutic spaces where community members can learn about various herbs, their uses, and cultivation techniques.

Spaces and Support

Start by scouting locations that are easily accessible to people in your community. Consider factors like accessibility for people with disabilities, traffic, and access to public transportation. It's crucial to scout multiple options to have a choice in your location.

Abandoned parks or lots often become the foundation for many community spaces. To advocate for your garden, talk to your city council and learn about zoning laws and local restrictions. There's power in numbers; the more people you connect with, the more you'll have to assist you in these tasks. For example, a fellow advocate might know a lawyer who can help with legal requirements.

You can also reach out to local businesses or professionals for assistance. Make sure to pitch the benefits of your garden, such as how it can help the local community, especially families and children. The garden could also benefit businesses by increasing traffic flow and offering fresh, locally-grown produce. Gather data and research to support your pitch, highlighting the positive effects of community gardens, like promoting healthy eating habits and providing green spaces for relaxation. Stress the potential economic benefits, such as job creation and increased property values. Build partnerships with schools, churches, and community organizations for support and resources. Be persistent and determined throughout the bureaucratic process to gain approval for your garden project.

Use social media to promote your garden and spread the word. Today's social media platforms reign supreme as the most efficient method to display your garden and engage with a vast audience. You can create dedicated pages or accounts on platforms such as Instagram, Facebook, or X to share pictures of your garden, gardening tips, and updates on any events or activities happening in your garden. If you need to become more familiar with social media, consider seeking assistance from younger or more tech-savvy individuals, such as college students or software engineers who can help you create a website. This will help generate interest and attract more visitors. Remember to articulate your mission clearly and have a signup sheet ready to gather more supporters. You can also use social media to collaborate with other gardening enthusiasts or influencers to cross-promote each other's gardens or organize joint events. Additionally, you can effectively target your desired audience and enhance the visibility of your garden through social media advertising.

With crowdfunding platforms like GoFundMe, you can easily reach out to others and seek financial assistance for your garden project. By creating a donation campaign, you can share your story, explain the purpose and vision of your garden, and request contributions from individuals who believe in your cause. Be sure to provide detailed information on how the funds will be utilized, whether for purchasing plants and seeds, maintaining the garden, or organizing educational programs. Sharing regular updates on your garden's progress and how the funds are used will help build trust and encourage more donations. Remember to express gratitude towards your supporters and acknowledge their contributions to further strengthen the community around your garden.

Again, we want to emphasize the community aspect of this. By working together and harnessing the power of numbers, you can expedite getting these things off the ground, ensuring a solid foundation of support for your garden.

Planning

With a few options in mind on the locations, you can start vetting them to see which is ideal for your community garden. You'll need to consider those factors we discussed in setting up your home garden, including hours of sunlight, water access, and soil quality, as well as additional factors such as safety and security. Let's go over these in a little more detail.

Once you have a few locations, you can begin vetting them to determine which is perfect for your community garden. You'll need to consider those factors we discussed in setting up your home garden, including sunlight, water, and soil, as well as additional factors such as safety and security. Let's go over these in a little more detail.

When vetting potential locations for your community garden, assessing the amount of sunlight each site receives is essential. Look for areas that receive at least six hours of direct sunlight per day, as this is crucial for the healthy growth of most plants.

You'll want to be sure you have water sources nearby. Access to water is essential for irrigation purposes, so ensure there is a convenient water supply or the possibility of installing irrigation systems.

Evaluating the soil quality is another vital factor. Conduct soil tests to determine its fertility, drainage, and composition, as this will affect the success of your garden.

Safety and Security

Safety and security should also be taken into account. You won't be just gardening for yourself but for people of all ages, backgrounds, and varying abilities. Watch out for hazards; consider families with children or pets when checking for potential risks.

Look for locations that are well-lit, easily accessible, and have low risks of vandalism or theft. Consider proximity to residential areas or public spaces, as this can enhance the sense of community and encourage participation. Lastly, consult local authorities and obtain any permits or permissions required to establish a community garden in the selected location.

Creating a Garden of Inclusion and Equality

Establish a tone for your garden by making acceptance and respect for all people a foundational principle. Our world is filled with conflicting views, so creating an open community where everyone feels included and valued is essential. Politics and religion are sensitive topics, and while people should be free to express their views, it must be done respectfully. Implement a zero-tolerance policy for hate and discrimination, ensuring that all potential members are aware of it. Your garden should bring light to the community and foster togetherness, so address any problems promptly and diplomatically. Take care of the hearts and minds of your community, just as you do with your plants, and both will thrive.

Moving Forward

Consider organizing workshops and classes on herbal medicine that can promote knowledge sharing and skill development among community members. These workshops can cover herbal remedies, formulations, and sustainable harvesting practices.

Another idea could be to establish herbal apothecaries or dispensaries in community areas. These spaces would offer a wide range of herbal products and remedies, promoting natural alternatives for health and wellness. Additionally, organizing regular herb walks and nature hikes would enable community members to engage with the local plant life and learn about the various herbs that flourish in their environment.

Creating herbal community spaces also fosters inclusivity and diversity, ensuring that these spaces welcome people from different backgrounds and experiences. Collaborating with local herbalists, healers, and indigenous communities can bring a wealth of knowledge and cultural perspectives to these spaces. Lastly, hosting community events such as herbal festivals, markets, and gatherings can further promote the importance of herbalism and create a sense of camaraderie among community members interested in plant-based healing.

Case Study: A Community Transformed Through Shared Herbal Spaces

The "Herbal Haven" project in Hammersmith and Fulham, London, is an inspiring example of how shared herbal spaces can positively impact a community. The government-funded this initiative, and it ran from April 2010 to January 2011. The project focused on growing herbs and creating simple cosmetics, home remedies, and household products. It provided a unique learning platform where individuals of all ages could interact, share knowledge, and bond over gardening activities. Participants learned about herbs and transformed their harvest into practical herbal products, which gave them a sense of accomplishment and community spirit. This project highlights communal herbal gardens' significant role in bridging generational gaps and enhancing community well-being (Herbal Haven – Hammersmith Community Gardens Association, n.d.).

SUSTAINABLE HERBAL GARDENING PRACTICES

We must consider our environmental impact as we create our herbal gardens and look forward to their benefits. Just as our gardens take care of us, we must also take care of the more extensive garden of nature that surrounds us. This starts with making sure our gardening practices are eco-friendly.

Eco-friendly gardening means practicing sustainable and environmentally conscious methods of gardening that minimize harm to the planet. This includes avoiding chemical pesticides and fertilizers and opting for natural or organic alternatives. It also involves conserving water using efficient irrigation techniques like drip irrigation or collecting rainwater.

Eco-friendly gardening promotes biodiversity by using native plants, attracting beneficial insects and wildlife, and practicing waste reduction through composting and recycling. Overall, it aims to create a harmonious and sustainable ecosystem in the garden, benefiting both the environment and the gardener. Below, we've compiled a list of tips to make your herbal garden eco-friendly.

1. **Selection of Location and Containers:** Choose a sunny spot with well-draining soil for your garden. Use biodegradable or recycled containers instead of plastic, reducing waste and promoting sustainability.
2. **Water Conservation:** Select drought-tolerant herbs like rosemary, thyme, and lavender. Consider vertical

gardening for its water-conserving benefits. This approach maximizes space while minimizing water usage.

3. **Organic Fertilization:** Use organic compost as a natural fertilizer instead of chemical alternatives. This enriches the soil with nutrients while avoiding harmful chemicals.

4. **Companion Planting:** Implement companion planting strategies to improve garden health and reduce the need for fertilizers and pesticides. This method involves planting certain herbs together to benefit each other.

5. **Attracting Beneficial Insects:** Encouraging a diverse ecosystem is essential for the health of your garden. One way to achieve this is by attracting insects such as bees, butterflies, and ladybugs. These insects can help with pollination and pest control, leading to a more successful garden. Planting various flowers and herbs that attract these pollinators enhances biodiversity and supports a healthy garden.

6. **Sustainable Harvesting:** Harvest herbs at their peak flavor and aroma. Use different methods like drying or freezing to preserve them for later use, reducing waste and extending the usefulness of your garden.

7. **Soil Health and Native Plants:** Improve soil health using compost and mulch, and choose native plants that support local insects and wildlife. Native plants typically require less feeding and watering, making them a sustainable choice.

8. **Natural Pest Control:** To maintain a healthy ecosystem in your garden, use eco-friendly techniques like natural pest control methods and avoid harmful pesticides.

Implementing these eco-friendly approaches will help you create a productive herbal garden while benefiting the environment and overall health.

Anecdotes: Success Stories of Sustainable Herbal Gardens

This story is about a tea lover who succeeded in sustainable herbal gardening by growing herbs such as lavender and mint, which are perfect for making tea. They started with easy-to-harvest herbs and then expanded to include cilantro and rosemary for cooking. The gardener adapted their practices to suit the changing seasons, for example, misting the plants during winter to retain moisture, much like they needed warmth and sunlight during colder months. This anecdote reflects a mindful and sustainable approach to herbal gardening that promotes personal well-being and environmental consciousness (Curtis, 2023).

ADVOCACY AND SHARING THE HERBAL WISDOM

Herbal advocates have a crucial role in our health-conscious society today. They protect ancient wisdom and practice a holistic approach to well-being. Their mission goes beyond individual health, as they aim to educate and empower communities to embrace the advantages of herbal wisdom fully.

Advocacy in herbalism encompasses a range of activities, including hosting workshops and seminars, writing articles, and producing online content. These endeavors demystify herbal practices and make their knowledge more accessible to a broader audience. Herbal advocates frequently collaborate with community centers, schools, and health clinics to introduce herbal therapies as complementary to conventional medicine.

Advocates of herbal knowledge emphasize the importance of sustainable practices, using local herbs, and ethically sourcing plant materials. They encourage communities to explore the rich diversity of plants in their local environment and learn how to use these plants for culinary and medicinal purposes.

Herbal advocates understand the importance of connecting with nature and recognize that our well-being is intricately linked to the planet's health. They emphasize using sustainable practices in harvesting and cultivating herbs, promoting the preservation of biodiversity and the protection of natural habitats. By prioritizing sustainability, they help ensure that future generations will have access to the healing properties of plants.

In addition to promoting sustainable practices, herbal advocates also highlight the significance of self-care. They encourage individuals to take responsibility for their health and well-being by incorporating herbal remedies into their daily routines. By embracing the power of plants, individuals can proactively support their physical, emotional, and spiritual health. Herbal advocates guide how to incorporate herbs into diets, create herbal remedies, and cultivate mindfulness practices that promote overall wellness.

Furthermore, herbal advocates recognize the importance of community well-being. They foster a sense of connection and belonging by creating spaces for individuals to come together and share their experiences with herbs. Through workshops, classes, and community events, they create opportunities for learning, collaboration, and support. By building a strong herbal community, advocates empower individuals to take control of their health and inspire others to do the same.

As we've seen, herbal advocates have a multifaceted responsibility beyond sharing knowledge. They ignite a profound bond with nature, advocate for sustainable practices, prioritize self-care, and promote community well-being. Through their efforts, they empower individuals to actively participate in their journey towards health and wellness while fostering a deeper connection with the natural world and supporting the overall well-being of their communities.

Case Study: A Successful Herbal Advocacy Campaign and Its Impact

The American Botanical Council (ABC), also known as the Herbal Medicine Institute, is dedicated to enhancing public knowledge and responsible use of herbs and medicinal plants. ABC is a non-profit organization that focuses on research and education. They provide peer-reviewed resources such as periodicals, books, monographs, and online databases. They aim to deliver consumers and professionals reliable, scientifically backed, and traditionally-informed information. This helps them make informed decisions for healthier living and integrate medicinal plants into their practice and research. ABC's advocacy in the herbal domain positively impacts various sectors of society.

Conclusion

As we come to the end of our journey through *The Therapeutic Power of Herbal Gardening*, it's essential to take a moment to reflect on the countless ways in which this practice can enhance our lives.

Undoubtedly, gardening has a remarkable therapeutic effect on our physical and mental states. It has been proven to alleviate stress, anxiety, and depression, elevate mood and self-confidence, and enhance cognitive abilities. Gardening is also a great way to exercise, connect with nature, and engage in a meaningful and rewarding activity.

But the benefits of herbal gardening go far beyond our well-being. The cultivation and utilization of herbs allow us to promote our planet's well-being and long-term viability actively. Herbal gardening is a way to support biodiversity, reduce our carbon foot-print, and encourage healthier ecosystems.

Herbs are also a valuable resource for holistic healing. They have been used for thousands of years to treat various ailments, from headaches and digestive issues to skin and respiratory problems. By learning about the medicinal properties of different herbs and how to use them safely and effectively, we can take control of our health and well-being.

Throughout this book, we've explored many aspects of herbal gardening, from the scientific and traditional to the practical and creative. We've learned about the importance of soil health, the benefits of companion planting, and the different methods for propagating and harvesting herbs. We've also explored many ways to use herbs in cooking, crafting, and natural remedies.

But perhaps, most importantly, we've discovered the profound connection between gardening and our sense of well-being. Through gardening, we can find solace from our busy lives and foster a deep connection with the wonders of the natural world. It's a way to find peace and serenity in a chaotic and over-whelming world.

As we move forward from this journey, let us carry the lessons we've learned and the inspiration we've gained. Let us continue to explore the world of herbal gardening, experiment with new plants and techniques, and find joy and fulfillment. And let us never forget that the true value of gardening lies not just in the result but in the journey itself.

So, as you move forward, remember to take time for yourself and your garden. Whether it's a few minutes each day or a more extended period once a week, make sure to take the time to connect with your plants and the earth. Listen to the birds, feel the sun on your face, and breathe in the fragrant scents of your garden.

As you tend to your herbs, allow yourself to be fully present in the moment. Take pleasure in the simple act of weeding, watering, and pruning. Allow yourself to experiment with herbs, from cooking to crafting to natural remedies.

And finally, remember that gardening is a never-ending process of learning and discovery. Whether you're a seasoned gardener or a complete novice, there's always something new to learn and explore. So, embrace the journey, wherever it may take you, and let the therapeutic power of herbal gardening continue to enrich your life for many years.

Happy gardening! May your hands find solace in the earth, and may your heart find solace in the beauty surrounding you.

Glossary

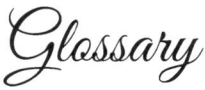

Adaptogen: A natural substance that aids the body in managing stress and maintaining internal stability.

Aeration: Refers to the process of adding air to soil to improve its overall health and fertility.

Advocacy: The act of publicly supporting a particular cause or policy.

Ailments: Illnesses or health problems.

Alchemy: The medieval predecessor to chemistry, centered on the supposed transmutation of substances.

Antioxidants: Molecules that prevent the oxidation of other molecules.

Aromatic: Refers to the pleasant scent or smell of a plant or other natural substance.

Aromatherapy: The use of aromatic plant oils to promote physical and psychological well-being.

Ayurvedic: Refers to a traditional system of medicine originating in India.

Biodiversity: Describes the existence of diverse plant and animal species in a specific habitat.

Cultivate: To grow or tend to plants to produce food or other resources.

Derivatives: Products derived from a particular source, such as a plant or mineral.

Ergonomically: Refers to equipment and devices designed to minimize discomfort and maximize efficiency.

Fertilizer: A substance added to soil to provide essential nutrients to plants.

Herbalists: Practitioners who use plants and herbs for medicinal purposes.

Holistic: Relating to the whole, considering the complete system rather than individual parts.

Horticulture: The science of cultivating plants.

Infusion is steeping a plant or other substance in a liquid, such as water or oil, to extract its beneficial properties.

Medicinal: Relating to the treatment of illness or disease through medical means.

Metabolic: Describes the biochemical reactions that sustain life in living organisms.

Mindfulness is the practice of being present and aware in the moment and is often used in gardening to connect with nature.

Mysticism: A religious or spiritual belief that involves a direct, personal experience of the divine.

Nurture: Caring for and promoting the growth and development of plants and other living organisms.

Oasis: Refers to a small, isolated area of vegetation in an otherwise arid or desert-like environment.

Oxidative: Refers to chemical reactions that involve the transfer of electrons.

pH level: A measurement of a substance's acidity or alkalinity. A pH tester is a tool used to measure the pH levels in soil and other materials.

Permeates: To spread or diffuse throughout a substance or environment.

Practitioners: Professionals who practice a particular profession, such as medicine, law, or therapy.

Prune: To trim away unnecessary or dead parts of a plant to promote growth and health.

Rehydrate: To restore the body's fluid levels by drinking water or other liquids.

Rejuvenation: The act of renewing or restoring something.

Salve: An ointment or balm used to soothe or heal the skin.

Soil fertility: The capability of soil to provide essential nutrients to plants.

Sowing: Planting seeds in soil or other growing medium to start a new plant.

Stewardship: The responsible management and care of something.

Supplements: Products, such as vitamins or minerals, are taken to supplement or enhance a person's diet.

Sustainability: The ability to maintain or support something over a long period.

Symbiotic: Refers to the interaction between two or more different organisms that benefits all parties involved.

Therapeutic: Refers to treating disease or illness and the benefits to the mind and body.

Tincture: The extract obtained from a plant or natural substance using alcohol.

Vermiculite: A common soil amendment made of mineral substance to improve drainage and aeration.

Waterlogging refers to the condition of soil oversaturated with water, which can damage plants and inhibit their growth.

Homemade Herbal Delights From My Garden

Dedicate this notepad section to capturing all the amazing homemade herbal creations you craft from your garden's bounty! Use this space to jot down recipes, track results, and personalize your herbal journey.

RECIPE:

- **Name:**
- **Date:**
- **Herbs Used: (List the specific herbs and their quantities)**

- **Other Ingredients: (Additional ingredients)**

- **Instructions: (Write the step-by-step process)**

- Notes: (Capture any observations, adjustments, or personalization you made)

RESULTS:

- Effects: (Describe the observed effects of the recipe, e.g., calming, energizing, relief for specific symptoms)

- Feedback: (Share your personal experience and enjoyment of the recipe)

- Adjustments: (Note any changes you'd make for the next time)

RECIPE:

- Name:
- Date:
- Herbs Used:

- Other Ingredients:

- Instructions:

- Notes:

RESULTS:

- Effects:

- Feedback:

- Adjustments:

RECIPE:

- Name:
- Date:
- Herbs Used:

- Other Ingredients:

- Instructions:

- Notes:

RESULTS:

- Effects:

- Feedback:

- Adjustments:

My Herbal Sanctuary: A Garden Journal

This section of your notepad invites you to delve deeper into the vibrant world of your herbal garden. Use this space to capture your observations, record insights, and track the growth and magic of your green companions.

HERB SPOTLIGHT:

Name: (Herb Name)

Date Planted:

Location: (Bed, pot, etc.)

Appearance: (Leaf shape, color, etc.)

Uses: (Culinary, medicinal, ailment, etc.)

Notes: (Interesting facts, personal observations, etc.)

Growth Tracker:

- Date:

- Height:

- Number of Leaves:

- Flowering/Fruiting: (Yes/No)

- Notes: (Any changes, observations, etc.)

Harvest Log:

- Date:

- Part Harvested: (Leaves, flowers, etc.)

- Quantity:

- Use: (Fresh, dried, etc.)

- Notes: (Successes, challenges, etc.)

Growth Tracker:

- Date:

- Height:

- Number of Leaves:

- Flowering/Fruiting:

- Notes:

Harvest Log:

- Date:

- Part Harvested:

- Quantity:

- Use:

- Notes:

Growth Tracker:

- Date:

- Height:

- Number of Leaves:

- Flowering/Fruiting:

- Notes:

Harvest Log:

- Date:

- Part Harvested:

- Quantity:

- Use:

- **Notes:**

References

5 Herbs You Can Grow with Mental Health Benefits. (2022, September 22). Heather LeGuilloux / Mental Health Blogger. https://www.heatherleguilloux.ca/blog/5-herbs-you-can-grow-with-mental-health-benefits

ABC Herbalgram Website. (n.d.). Www.herbalgram.org. Retrieved January 31, 2024, from https://www.herbalgram.org/about-us/

Batke, S. (2023, April 17). *How plants can change your state of mind.* The Conversation. https://theconversation.com/how-plants-can-change-your-state-of-mind-198010

breeshop. (2019, September 6). *Soil Healing: An Inner & Outer Journey.* Howard Creek Ranch. https://www.howardcreekranch.com/2019/09/06/soil-healing-an-inner-outer-journey/

Carrey, J. (n.d.). *The Divine Feminine Art of Flower Essence Therapy: Emotional Healing 101 (Part 1).* Jana Carrey Healing || Ancient Alchemy for Modern Beings®. Retrieved January 30, 2024, from https://www.janacarrey.com/journal/2019/9/5/an-introduction-to-flower-essences-one-of-the-most-powerful-emotional-healing-tools-on-the-planet

Chiocca, R. (2023, October 18). *Therapeutic Gardens: Healing Stories from the World of Horticulture.* Robert Chiocca. https://robertchiocca.com/2023/10/18/therapeutic-gardens-healing-stories-from-the-world-of-horticulture/

Clegg, B. (2013, August 13). *15 Herb Bouquets (And What They Symbolize!).* Theknot.com; The Knot. https://www.theknot.com/content/15-herb-bouquets-and-what-they-symbolize

Companion, H. (2001, July 1). *Natural healing Summertime herbs - Mother Earth Living.* Www.motherearthliving.com. https://www.motherearthliving.com/health-and-wellness/Natural-Healing-Summertime-Herbs/

Crossley, H. (2022, January 30). *We talk to experts about the advantages of getting outdoors and tending to nature.* Gardeningetc.com. https://www.gardeningetc.com/features/gardening-for-mental-health

Cultivating Health. (2022, December 14). *10 health benefits of meditation and how to focus on mindfulness.* Cultivating-Health. https://health.ucdavis.edu/blog/cultivating-health/10-health-benefits-of-meditation-and-how-to-focus-on-mindfulness-and-compassion/2022/12

Curtis, P. (2023, August 9). *Don't Overthink Gardening.* The Atlantic. https://www.theatlantic.com/science/archive/2023/08/gardening-beginning-principles/674962/

Devon. (2016, February 6). *Growing a Medicinal Herb Garden for Health & Wellness.* Nitty Gritty Life. https://nittygrittylife.com/creating-a-medicinal-herb-garden/

Dilger, C. (2023, November 3). *Here's How To Create a Wellness Centered Home, According to An Expert.* Home & Texture. https://homeandtexture.com/wellness-centered-home/

Fleckenstein, A., & MD. (2014, November 5). *16 Healing Herbs For The Most Amazing Bath Of Your Life.* Prevention. https://www.prevention.com/health/health-condi tions/a20472817/healing-herbs-to-use-in-a-bath/

Gagliano, M. (2017). The mind of plants: Thinking the unthinkable. *Communicative & Integrative Biology, 10*(2), e1288333. https://doi.org/10.1080/19420889.2017.1288333

Gardening for Mental Health | the Herb Garden. (2022, February 21). Herb Garden. https://herbgarden.ca/2022/02/21/gardening-for-mental-health/

Gladstar, R. (2014). Herbs for Common Ailments: How to Make and Use Herbal Remedies for Home Health Care. A Storey BASICS® Title. In *Amazon* (New edition). Storey Publishing, LLC. My Book

Gladstar, R. (2022, April 11). *Growing Awareness with Botanical Sanctuaries - The Science & Art of Herbalism.* Scienceandartofherbalism.com. https://scienceandartofherbal ism.com/growing-awareness-with-botanical-sanctuaries/

Herbal Haven — Hammersmith Community Gardens Association. (n.d.). Herbal Haven. Retrieved January 28, 2024, from https://hcga.org.uk/projects/herbal-haven/

Herbalism, W. (2023, October 4). *Spatial Alchemy: Changing Through Herbal Smoke - The Alchemist's Kitchen.* The Alchemist's Kitchen. https://wisdom.thealchemist skitchen.com/spatial-alchemy-changing-through-herbal-smoke/

Hruschak, K. (n.d.). *Unlock the Nutrition Potential: The Benefits of Growing Herbs for Your Loved Ones.* Aging Well Nutrition Services. Retrieved February 1, 2024, from https://www.agingwellnutrition.ca/blog/unlock-the-nutrition-potential-herbs

Jami. (2019, April 30). *Herb Garden Before and After + Updates Through the Seasons.* An Oregon Cottage. https://anoregoncottage.com/new-herb-garden-before-and-after/

Jamie. (2022, March 25). *The 6 Different Types Of Soil (All You Need To Know).* The Backyard Pros. https://thebackyardpros.com/types-of-soil/

Johnson, C. (2014, October 7). *Fall Harvest Activities for Horticultural Therapy | Chicago Botanic Garden.* Www.chicagobotanic.org. https://www.chicagobotanic.org/blog/ learning/fall_harvest_activities_horticultural_therapy

Koulivand, P. H., et al. (2013). Lavender and the Nervous System. Evidence-Based Complementary and Alternative Medicine.

Lasswell, I. (2019, September 21). *Aromatics in the Ancient World: History Of Aromatherapy | World History.* Worldhistory.us. https://worldhistory.us/general/ aromatics-in-the-ancient-world-history-of-aromatherapy.php

Leech, J. (2017, June 4). *10 Delicious Herbs and Spices With Powerful Health Benefits.*

Healthline. https://www.healthline.com/nutrition/10-healthy-herbs-and-spices#TOC_TITLE_HDR_3

Leone, M. (2021, June 21). *RITUALS OF ABUNDANCE for the Summer Solstice*. Anima Mundi Herbals. https://animamundiherbals.com/blogs/blog/rituals-of-abundance-for-the-summer-solstice

Lovelace, B. (2022, December 22). *No more stress in 2023? Americans aren't too optimistic about that*. NBC News. https://www.nbcnews.com/health/health-news/adults-say-expecting-stress-2023-survey-finds-rcna62580

McIntyre, E., Saliba, A. J., & Moran, C. C. (2015). Herbal medicine use in adults who experience anxiety: A qualitative exploration. *International Journal of Qualitative Studies on Health and Well-Being, 10*(1), 29275. https://doi.org/10.3402/qhw.v10.29275

Medicinals, T. (2021, April 9). *Herbal Bouquets*. Traditional Medicinals. https://ca.traditionalmedicinals.com/articles/herbal-bouquets/

Nichols, J. (2017, August 4). *How to Decorate With Herb Plants*. Love My Simple Home. https://www.lovemysimplehome.com/2016/09/decorating-with-herbs.html

Ortiz, P. (2023, January 17). *How to Make Potting Soil for Herbs — 5 Simple Steps*. House Grail. https://housegrail.com/how-to-make-potting-soil-for-herbs/#:

Petrovska, B. B. (2012). Historical review of medicinal plants' usage. *Pharmacognosy Reviews, 6*(11), 1-5. https://doi.org/10.4103/0973-7847.95849

Popham, S. (2019, October 9). *The Practice of Herbal Alchemy: An Interview with Master Alchemist Robert Bartlett*. The School of Evolutionary Herbalism. https://www.evolutionaryherbalism.com/2019/10/09/the-practice-of-herbal-alchemy/

Prasad, S., et al. (2014). Turmeric, the Golden Spice: From Traditional Medicine to Modern Medicine. In Herbal Medicine: Biomolecular and Clinical Aspects. 2nd edition. CRC Press/Taylor & Francis.

Schrum, C. (2018, May 30). *13 Natural Remedies for Common Ailments*. Experience Life. https://experiencelife.lifetime.life/article/13-natural-remedies-for-common-ailments/

Shah, S. A., et al. (2007). Evaluation of Echinacea for the Prevention and Treatment of the Common Cold: A Meta-Analysis. The Lancet Infectious Diseases.

Singh, N. (2023, November 30). *Embracing Serenity: Discovering Tranquility in Life's Serene Moments*. Medium. https://medium.com/@1993navjeet/embracing-serenity-discovering-tranquility-in-lifes-serene-moments-a66ec4ee17d6

Sky News. (2021, April 17). Gardening regularly improves mental and physical wellbeing, RHS study shows. Retrieved from https://news.sky.com/story/gardening-regularly-improves-mental-and-physical-wellbeing-rhs-study-shows-12287363

Summer Solstice Herbs & Flowers. (2023, June 21). Faith in Nature. https://www.faithinnature.co.uk/blogs/notes-on-nature/summer-solstice-herbs-and-flowers

The Emergency Doctor Who Teaches Herbal Medicine. (2019). *Restorative Medicine*

Digest. https://restorativemedicine.org/digest/emergency-doctor-teaches-herbal-medicine/

Tuff®C. F. &. (2017, June 22). *Aromatic bliss – Master the art of home aromatherapy! - Cascades.* Cascades Fluff & Tuff. https://www.cascadesflufftuff.com/en/blog/posts/2017/june/aromatic-bliss-master-the-art-of-aromatherapy

Van Sloun, N. (2015, November 28). *Natural Remedies for Everyday Illnesses.* Www.allinahealth.org. https://www.allinahealth.org/healthysetgo/heal/natural-remedies-for-everyday-illnesses

Voiles, S. (n.d.). *Ritual Bath.* Sarah K Voiles. Retrieved January 28, 2024, from https://www.sarahkvoiles.com/blog/ritual-bath

Wee JJ, Mee Park K, Chung AS. Biological Activities of Ginseng and Its Application to Human Health. In: Benzie IFF, Wachtel-Galor S, editors. Herbal Medicine: Biomolecular and Clinical Aspects. 2nd edition. Boca Raton (FL): CRC Press/Taylor & Francis; 2011. Chapter 8. Available from: https://www.ncbi.nlm.nih.gov/books/NBK92776/

Weides, A. (2022, November 12). *What Is a Meditation Garden? • Gardenary.* Gardenary. https://www.gardenary.com/blog/what-is-a-meditation-garden

Winfield, A. (2023, June 29). *Magical plants of the Summer Solstice – University of Bristol Botanic Garden.* Botanic-Garden.bristol.ac.uk. https://botanic-garden.bristol.ac.uk/2023/06/29/3155/

Woman, G. (2024, January 8). *Seeds of Change: Caroline's Journey from Herbal Gardens to Global Wellbeing Advocate.* Global Woman Magazine. https://globalwoman magazine.com/seeds-of-change-carolines-journey-from-herbal-gardens-to-global-wellbeing-advocate/

Wu, C. (2020, November 12). *Case Studies on Children in Community Gardens and Gardening with Children.* Each Green Corner. Retrieved February 18, 2024, from /

Made in the USA
Columbia, SC
22 June 2025

59715408R00109